take charge of your
beauty

Insider Tips for *Restoring and Enhancing*
Your Natural Beauty without Surgery

LINDA RANK

Website: www.skinmedxcenter.com

Email: rank@skinmedxcenter.com

Phone: 949-836-8120

Ordering Information: Quantity sales. Special discounts are available on multiple purchases by corporations, associations, and others.

Address:

For details, contact the "Special Sales Department" at the address above.

Take Charge of Your Beauty, Linda Rank–1st edition, 2017

Book Layout: © 2017 Evolve Global Publishing www.evolveglobalpublishing.com

ISBN: 978-1-64136-492-8 (Paperback)

ISBN: 978-1-64136-493-5 (Hardcover)

ISBN-13: 978-1977516770 (Createspace)

ISBN-10: 1977516777 (Createspace)

ISBN: (Smashwords)

ASIN: B071GQ15Q4 (Amazon Kindle)

This book is available on Barnes & Noble, Kobo, Apple iBooks (digital)

Table of Contents

About the Author

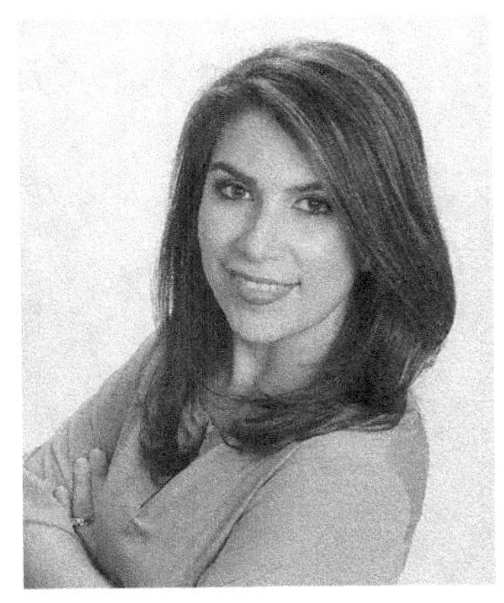

Linda Rank, PA-C studied the Physician Assistant Program at the Charles R. Drew University School of Medicine and Science in Los Angeles after she completed a Bachelor of Arts Degree in Psychology at the University of California, Santa Cruz. She has been specializing in dermatology since 2001, and she maintains Certification from the National Board of Medical Examiners.

As a personable, knowledgeable, and competent Physician Assistant, Linda has a broad range of medical dermatology experience, and she is qualified to order and interpret laboratory test results and write prescriptions.

Linda has experience with successfully treating patients of all ages and for a wide range of skin conditions. The scope of her dermatology practice traverses the diagnosis and treatment of skin disorders, skin cancer examinations, and treatment of skin cancers, in addition to an extensive range of cosmetic procedures. She has over 15 years of experience working with Botox, dermal fillers, laser treatments, and many other cosmetic procedures.

Linda is a current member of the American Academy of Physician Assistants, California Academy of Physician Assistants and Society of Dermatology Physician Assistants.

Introduction

As a young girl, I remember seeing hundreds of plastic bottles of skin lotion in my mother's closet. It was my job to assist her to fill them up and apply labels to each bottle. At the time, I didn't really understand exactly what I was doing, although I knew that my mom sold these lotions to women to make them pretty. I remember visiting her at the salon where she worked; I did my homework there while she used her skills to help women look better. She was an esthetician who did facials, waxing, eyebrows, and skin care. This was during the 1980s when there was no Facebook, no Amazon, and no Internet—just magazines that told women about beauty and how to both achieve and preserve their beauty.

My mom listened to the stories of women who wanted to retain their looks or improve their appearance, and she had her own story to tell as well. After 25 years, she found herself divorced, with no career or skills. Nevertheless, a single mother of three dependent children, she needed to find a way to support herself and her family. The stories of her clients often intertwined with the stories of her own life. I'm not exactly sure why she got into skin care, but she definitely found her calling in this field. Clients warmed to her, and she easily shared in their stories. They trusted the woman with the beautiful skin. Her clients were from the San Fernando Valley, and mostly from the south side of Ventura Boulevard. They included stay-at-home wives and moms, professional women, and women in the entertainment business. She worked in Calabasas, now home of the Kardashians, and she often came home with stories about her customers' lives. At that time, her stories didn't mean much to me because I was preoccupied with my teenage life. I do remember though that she gave us regular advice about beauty. Some of the messages I recall are:

"Your looks only last so long."

"Looks are important."

"Don't depend on anyone."

"Don't let yourself go."

She always encouraged my sisters and me to pursue a career so that we could take care of ourselves. While her spoken messages told me to always wear sunscreen and blush, her deeper messages made a lasting impression on me though I never realized how profoundly they would impact me later in life.

Looking back, I'm not exactly sure how my mom did it, but her messages had an enduring impact on all of us. All three of her girls became professionals in the medical field, and most certainly, all of us are independent women who take charge of our own lives. I have spent a lifetime listening to my mother's stories, and as the youngest of three girls in my family, I have developed into a quiet observer both in my personal life and in my medical career. Women are great storytellers. If you listen carefully enough, you can learn a lot from women about life, mistakes, heroes, and even a lot about yourself, including how to love yourself.

I graduated from the University of California at Santa Cruz with a degree in psychology. I decided to put aside my dreams of being a therapist and pursued a career in medicine. In 2001, I became a physician assistant. I never contemplated a career in dermatology, but as fate would have it, I followed the road of least resistance, and many doors opened for me. I was offered a part-time, temporary position to train with a dermatologist to fill a staffing vacancy while another doctor was on maternity leave. At this time, dermatology was not the glamorous speciality it has become today. I won't lie; it was much less stressful than urgent care or a walk-in clinic. There were many cases of skin cancer, rashes, acne, itchiness, and all manner of ailments to do with hair, skin, and nails.

I remember attending a training session on something called Botox. It was a "toxin to freeze your face" and get rid of wrinkles. At the time, I was in my mid-twenties, and I remember thinking to myself that I had no interest whatsoever in injecting this stuff, and I never imagined I would need it. I was going to age gracefully. I wanted to practice medicine and help people. But, there was a sort of revolution going on.

Faster than anyone could have predicted, Botox became the jewel in the crown of aesthetic medicine! Every patient in the clinic was asking me about it; every medical provider outside of the dermatology speciality was curious and sceptical about it. At every social event I attended, I was surrounded by women asking about "the secret of youth"—Botox.

Eventually, Botox was approved, and a few years later, it became a household word. I changed my mind about it when I saw some really impressive results. After years of injecting both Botox and dermal fillers, then adding lasers to my repertoire, my experience sharpened me, and my views about the world of aesthetics evolved.

Looking back at my 15 years in dermatology, I realized that I never really moved far from psychology, after all. Everyone on the planet, whether it's a man, a woman, young, old, professional, or a stay-at-home mom, has a story. I learned to listen to these as my mother listened to her clients years ago because listening is very much a part of the healing I offer.

Book Overview

This book provides an informative and comprehensive overview of non-invasive cosmetic procedures that are currently used in contemporary dermatology, and it is intended as a guide to introduce readers to the plethora of options that have now reached the market, all of which are designed to enhance, restore, and rejuvenate your appearance, with minimal downtime and impressive results.

The book begins with discussing why you should take care of your beauty now, and it also provides an overview of some of the newest innovations in cosmetic dermatology. discuss the fascinating science of beauty, based on universal mathematical principles and contemporary research findings.

Sun protection is discussed with priority because it remains the number one cause of premature aging, so I have dedicated an entire chapter to sun protection early in the book to provide readers with a thorough education about what they need to know and exactly what they need to be doing in regards to protecting their skin from the sun's harmful ultraviolet rays. There is an additional chapter about skincare, which provides thorough guidelines about what skincare products readers should be using for their skin type. The author also discusses specific types of cosmetic concerns and the non-invasive options that are currently available to address each type of skin concern. This discussion also specifies procedures that might be useful for patients according to their age (from their twenties to into their fifties, and beyond).

Subsequent chapters provide a detaie detailed explanation of Botox, dermal Fillers and several noninvasive procedures such as lasers, photofacials and chemical peels. Also reviewed are newer procedures, such as micro-needling, Prp PRP (Platlelet Rich Plasma) and non-invasive fat removal procedures. In some detail she discusses their uses, limitations, contraindications, advantages, what to expect during treatment, and discussions of each type of treatment. The book also addresses important questions for readers to ask their skincare specialists before committing to any procedure.

The book concludes with a series of frequently asked questions, and finally, a discussion about the future of cosmetic dermatology.

CHAPTER ONE

Why You Should Take Care of Your Beauty Now!

Let's face it: All of us want to look out best. When clients first come to see me, they will often say: "I wish these wrinkles would go away!" or "I wish I looked like I did ten years ago!" We all wish for similar things. So, what is the real problem?

Over the years, I have had a lot of patients who have come to me to help them both restore and maintain their beauty. Some of these women are in their seventies and eighties. In fact, I have worked with numerous 70- and 80-year-old ladies who have looked after themselves impeccably over the years and who are still entering beauty pageants—they look amazing!

I have had other, very busy ladies, newly divorced ladies, single mothers, ladies who have careers, and ladies of teenage children whose middle age has slowly crept up on them, and for the first time in many years, they have truly seen themselves in the mirror—to their horror, they realize they have lost the youthful, unlined appearance they had ten or fifteen years ago. In each one of these cases, I have been in the position to offer these ladies safe and effective solutions to both enhance and restore their beauty, and it is an utter privilege and honor to witness the overall substantial improvements in their confidence and well-being.

In my experience, the psychological benefits of beauty enhancement are far-reaching. They include increased self-esteem, overcoming feelings of helplessness, feeling more in control of their lives, becoming more sociable and outgoing, increased happiness, feeling more attractive, feeling good when looking in the mirror, feeling younger, as well as increased motivation to adopt other healthful lifestyle practices. With benefits like these, who wouldn't want to do everything they can to enhance their beauty?

The problem is that as we age, our skin loses the elasticity that it is needed for it to hold its shape. So, things like wrinkles, droopy eyelids and less volume in your cheeks might make you look more tired, worried, or even worse—older than your actual age. Essentially, as you get older, the dead cells of your skin start to accumulate, which can make the complexion become dull and uneven in tone. Thankfully, with advancements in treatments and procedures, our wishes can be granted with minimum effort, minimal recovery, and longer-lasting results.

Aging: The Very Unpopular Process of Getting Older

We all know we are, by and large, living longer than our ancestors, but what are the driving forces of aging and what impact does that have on our skin? Moreover, what additional measures can we take to ensure that we protect our largest organ to help keep it looking radiant? Aging is a gradual process that is connected to changes that affect the appearance, characteristics, and function of the skin. It is a synergistic effect of genetic, lifestyle, dietary, and environmental factors, which can be defined as intrinsic or chronological factors versus extrinsic or photoaging factors. As the name suggests, intrinsic factors are internal physiological changes, whereas extrinsic factors are external that happen synergistically to cause visible signs of aging.

Intrinsic/Chronological Factors: During our mid-twenties, collagen production slows down and the elastin, which gives the skin its "snap back" diminishes, and at the same time, the cycle of cell renewal slows down. Our genetic makeup largely determines the speed of this process.

Here are a few of the signs of intrinsic aging:

Some fine wrinkles due to changes in the dermis (deep layer of skin). Your skin may become slack as the loss of elastin in the skin causes the skin to hang loosely. Your skin might become itchy, or parts of your skin might be rougher or more course than usual. The reduction of fatty tissue in the cheeks, temples, chin, nose, and eye area may result in looser, sunken, or darker skin.

Unfortunately, there are a lot more!

Extrinsic/Photoaging: Extrinsic aging occurs due to ever-increasing age-advancing and critically destructive environmental pollution. Our skin is under constant assault by air- and water-borne elements that continuously degrade the condition of our skin and general well-being, otherwise known as environmental stress. Two of the key factors are:

1. Environmental Pollution/Debris Pollution: This refers to the release of environmental contaminants. The major forms of pollution include air pollution and the release of chemicals and particulates into the atmosphere. The presence of chemical, mineral, radioactive, or biological substances that alter/attack our natural environmental defense system (which, over time, result in the deterioration of the condition of our skin) heavily contribute to aging.

2. UV Radiation: This is a slow process that results from chronic and/or acute exposure to solar UV. It occurs for several decades before it becomes obvious. The degree of photoaging you will experience is determined by your skin type and by your total sun exposure over the course of your life. All doses of ultraviolet radiation (UVR) contribute to photoaging.

Arguably, exposure to sunlight is the single biggest felon. Sunlight most commonly affects the face, chest, arms, hands, and legs. Even a few minutes of UV exposure per day over the course of your life will contribute to the visible signs of photoaging. Those of you with fair skin will develop more signs of photoaging faster than those with dark skin. UV radiation in sunlight damages the elastin and collagen fibers in the skin. This damage may not show in your younger years, but it will later in life.

Common Signs of Photoaging:

- Freckles or age spots
- Rough and leathery skin
- Wrinkles (both fine lines and coarse wrinkles)
- A blotchier complexion
- Skin cancer

Good Skincare Is Critical Because People Are Living Longer and Working Longer

Today, we are not only living longer, but we are also working longer. We have more stress in our lives, but many of us are time-poor, which leads to poor lifestyle choices that have negative consequences for our entire physiology, and which are then reflected in our skin! There are three lifestyle factors that have been well-documented, which are serious culprits when it comes to progressing the signs of aging, causing us to look far older than our years. I will discuss each of these briefly.

Diet

As I am sure you are already aware, poor nutrition will contribute to looking older and overall skin aging. A diet that is low in fresh fruit and vegetables, high in processed food, and a habit of replacing water for coffee or sugary sodas (which are diuretics) may well accelerate the aging process.

Smoking

Let's face it, smokers generally develop face wrinkles far earlier than nonsmokers. As you are likely aware, smoking reduces blood flow to the skin, which then causes damage to the tissues (collagen and elastin), which help keep skin looking young. If we look at the complexion of people who have smoked for a number of years, the complexion is dull and lackluster. Of course, smoking may also increase the risk of skin cancers of both the skin and lips, and in addition, smoking is likely to accelerate the damage caused by sun exposure. The constant-puckering of the lips while smoking will substantially increase the wrinkles around the mouth, which ensures looking older!

Alcohol

Poor skin texture and wrinkles caused by dehydration can result from drinking too much alcohol. Alcohol dehydrates your body generally, including the skin, and will deprive the skin of vital vitamins and nutrients. Over time, alcohol can have other, more permanent, damaging effects on your skin. Facial redness, flushing, and rosacea are among possible effects of excessive alcohol consumption. Increased blushing and blotching, if untreated, can eventually lead to facial scarring, which can become severe and very difficult to treat.

What Non-invasive Procedures Can Restore My Skin?

As non-invasive procedures have become increasingly commonplace, the prices have dropped, and they are now accessible to most people. Although we want to look better, we don't want anyone to know what we have had done—we just want them to say, "Wow; you look great!"

It goes without saying that there is no single solution to looking your best that will suit everyone, and not every procedure will be right for every problem. The best beauty enhancement procedures for you will very much depend on your skin type, lifestyle, and general health. Naturally, you also need to consider your budget, the amount of time you have, and the level of discomfort you're willing to accept.

I cannot emphasize enough how important it is to ask plenty of questions before any treatment, so keep in mind that you don't need something like a facelift to smooth wrinkles around your mouth or eyes. Your objective is to walk out of the clinic looking less tired, more energetic, and youthful—like your younger self. Once you find a specialist you are comfortable with, your specialist can advise you about the best options for you to achieve what you want. Depending on what you are wanting, your specialist may even combine procedures as part of an ongoing treatment plan–this is an option that I offer all my clients!

Keep This In Mind

There's no such thing as a "non-surgical facelift." Usually, non-surgical procedures are targeted for people between 30–60 years old, who have reasonably good skin and protect it from the sun. Some procedures can can involve some pain, so you may need a recovery period at home. These procedures are not a surgical facelift. The results won't be as long-lasting, and repeated treatments may possibly end up exceeding the cost of a surgical facelift. You get what you pay for: Practitioners who offer discounts may be under-trained and lack the experience necessary for evaluations, and more importantly, for performing the procedure safely. There are no guarantees with cosmetic physicians either, but the odds of a safe and effective procedure are better if you choose someone with the necessary skills, experience, and credentials. There are risks with all procedures and treatments: There is nothing on the market at present that is completely risk-free.

Examples of Noninvasive Treatments Available

- Botox
- Dermal fillers
- Chemical peel
- Dermal rolling
- Microdermabrasion
- Radio frequency
- Intense pulsed light (IPL)

Make Sure You Ask

- How long it will take and what is involved?
- What you should expect immediately after the procedure
- Whether you will need to take time off work due to any side-effects
- What the costs of the procedure are, including aftercare and the cost of take-home skincare products, etc.
- Approximately how many sessions you will need to see results
- If you need more than one session, whether there is a package available
- If you don't use all the sessions, whether you get a refund.
- If something goes wrong, would they be able to help you and how?

Be cautious when reading reviews because results can be subjective and based on expectation rather than the procedure itself, operator error, or outdated technology. Be mindful that some procedures take some time to have optimal effects.

There is a plethora of before-and-after photos highlighting the different treatments when searching online, but be mindful that advertisers tend to show optimal rather than typical outcomes. Also, be mindful that the treatment is only as good as the specialist who is performing it and the products that they use. Make sure you ask the questions because there are risks involved. So, to be safe, do your research.

It Is Far Better to Be Proactive than Reactive

So, we all agree, it is far better to be proactive than feeling you need to be reactive! Protecting   the skin is always important, and this is particularly so during the summer months. Despite what marketing companies tell us, nothing can completely reverse the sun damage that is done during our youth. The good news though is that you can prevent the skin from becoming more damaged by staying out of the sun and/or by protecting yourself as much as possible.

There are certainly things that you can change about your lifestyle to preserve the condition of your skin. Stopping smoking, reducing your alcohol intake, and replacing processed foods with plenty of fruit and vegetables will go a long way towards preserving your skin.

We need to all take responsibility and ensure that we care for our skin, which is not only our largest organ, but our first line of defense to protect us from environmental stressors. Unfortunately, no one else is going to do this for you. This book will provide you with thorough insight, knowledge, and advice to help you put your best face forward. Your face will represent you, and with a longer life and work expectancy, there will be a time that you will care.

There is no question that aging is a complex process that involves both intrinsic and external factors, but thankfully, aging is not a disease: It is a perfectly normal process that happens to everyone. Nevertheless, the more prepared and educated we are, the healthier our skin and the better we look!

CHAPTER TWO

The Science of Beauty

Beauty Is in the Phi of the Beholder

It is widely accepted that beauty is defined by culture, and what is perceived as beautiful is a by-product of cultural and societal norms. Scientists now believe that our perception of physical beauty is actually hardwired for humans, and human perception of beauty has much to do with numbers. These numbers are referred to as the Golden Ratio (phi), and these ratios can be found throughout nature. In beauty, these numbers (ratios) are reflected in the proportions of a person's face. Evidence shows that the closer facial proportions are to the Golden Ratio, the more attractive the face is perceived across all races, cultures, and historical eras.

What Is the Golden Ratio?

The Greek philosopher Phidias (480BC–430BC) believed there was a numerical code of beauty in the universe. Phidias observed that all plants and animals grow in a precise manner and adhere to universal geometric patterns. The Greeks believed that the patterns were based on a geometrical ratio called the Golden Ratio.

The Golden Ratio is a special number that is found by dividing a line into two parts so that the longer part divided by the smaller part is also equal to the whole length divided by the longer part. This number is called phi, (after the Greek philosopher, Phidias).

This is the symbol for phi: uppercase to the left and lowercase on the right:

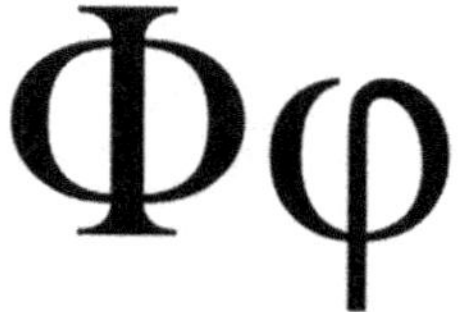

Below is the formula for calculating the Golden Ratio:

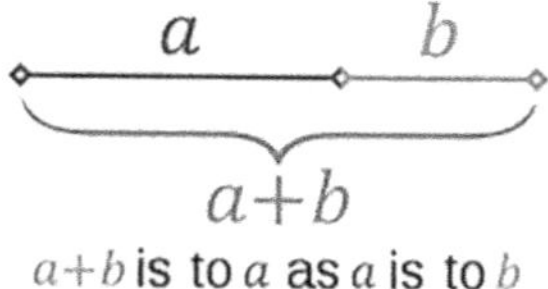

Phi can be observed throughout the universe. Phi is reflected in the proportions of the human body, plants, DNA, the solar system, art and music, population growth, the stock market, and the Bible.

Similarly, buildings are more attractive if the proportions adhere to the Golden Ratio. The same ratio has been used throughout history by architects and artists to produce objects of great beauty, like Michelangelo's David, the Greek temples, and the pyramids in Egypt. The Golden Ratio also occurs throughout nature, and it is observed in many of the beautiful patterns that we see in flowers, pinecones, and animals.

So, what has mathematics got to do with beauty? History has shown us that mathematics and beauty are closely intertwined. Physical attraction depends on ratio. Our attraction to another person's body increases if that body is symmetrical and in proportion. Likewise, if a face is in proportion, we are more likely to notice it and find it beautiful. Leonardo da Vinci's drawings of the human body emphasized proportion. The ratio in the Vitruvian Man image approximates the Golden Ratio.

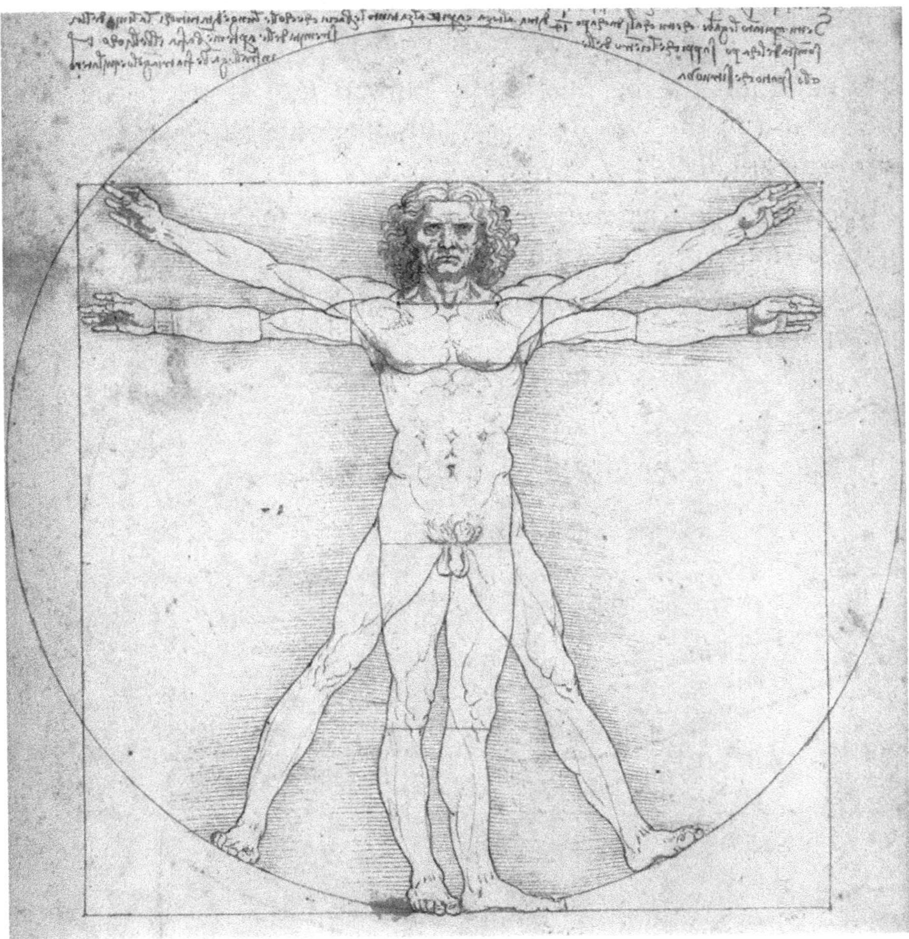

It is often assumed that the ratio of the radius of the circle to the side length of the square (i.e., the height of the Vitruvian Man) adheres to the Golden Ratio.

You can test this yourself: Measure the distance from the floor to your navel and then measure from your navel to your head. If you are well-proportioned, your ratio would be 1:1.618! This ratio is evident across the entire human body.

Therefore, the beauty of the human face is defined as the proportion of the two main measurements of the face, vertically and horizontally.

Vertically: the distance between the pupils and mouth in relation to the distance of the hairline to the chin.

Horizontally: the distance between the pupils in relation to the width of the face.

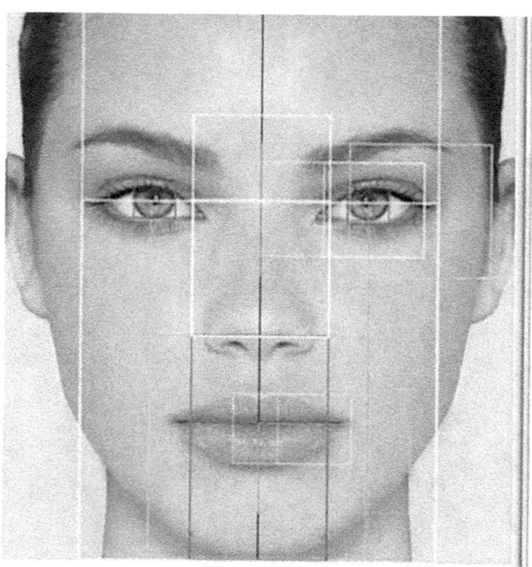
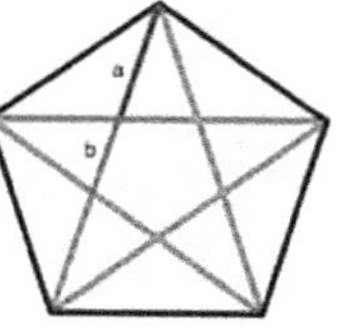

Dr. Stephen Marquardt, a plastic surgeon who performs surgeries on disfigured faces, has studied the science of beauty for many years to improve the results for his patients. He performed cross-cultural surveys on beauty and found that all groups had the same perceptions of facial beauty. He studied the human face from ancient times to the modern day, and discovered that beauty is not only related to phi, but that it is universally defined for both genders and for all races, cultures, and eras.

The template of beauty is found in the universal rules of phi, and the patterns of beauty can be measured with triangles and pentagons. He built a mask using these geometric proportions and learned that the closer a face matches them, the more that face will be perceived as beautiful.

He contends that we have triangles in the face, including in the width of the nose or profile of the nose, and that the smile is a pentagon consisting of multiple triangles. In the face, the sides of the triangle and the width of the base are often 1:1.6182, and these triangles form a pentagon using these measurements. A smile creates a pentagon between the nose, lips, chin, and jawline. Dr. Marquardt is able to utilize his mask of ratios when reconstructing faces with deformities. The face mask that Dr. Marquardt designed applies cross culturally.

There's a good reason why we perceive a warm smile as beautiful rather than the cold look of anger, arrogance, or contempt. The human face conforms most closely to phi proportions when we smile. An important caveat of these observations is that symmetry in the face does not necessarily equate to beauty. Many, if not most, faces that are perceived as beautiful are usually not even close to having perfect symmetry between the left and right sides. In fact, perfect symmetry tends to result in a face that appears unnatural, unanimated, or robot-like.

Beauty Through the Years

Beauty changes as we age. Baby beauty differs from adult beauty. Babies are generally perceived as attractive with their big eyes, full cheeks, and rosy lips all scrunched together. As we age, these same features are still considered attractive, but there are some differences. For female attractiveness, the two most common predictors are youth and health. Characteristics, like clear skin and full lips, contribute to attractiveness.

The age range when beauty peaks for women is between the ages of 14 and 24. According to Dr. Marquardt, what elevates some young women to have model-level beauty is having attributes of an adult beautiful face together with features of a beautiful baby face. Defining features of female beauty are high cheekbones, a nice forehead, a defined jawline, and an aligned nose, combined with the baby features of a slightly retruded chin, a strong Cupid's bow mouth, along with the short upper lip of a baby.

Another theory about the science of beauty is believed to stem from evolution and animal-like drives, which are thought to be influenced by the instinct to mate. As far back as thousands of years ago, there is evidence that humans had some understanding about human beauty. Human beings have been using makeup now for over 4,000 years! Ancient Egyptian women used many of the same techniques used today to enhance their beauty, like outlining their eyes with kohl. Makeup has always been used to cover up skin discolorations and enhance and contour lips and eyes.

A popular trend in eye makeup is to create "bedroom eyes." What are they and why are they considered beautiful? Well, this goes back to the primal instinct to mate; in the moments before an orgasm, the muscle of the upper eyelid relaxes, causing it to droop slightly, so bedroom eye makeup subconsciously reminds us of mating. Lipstick also has similar sexual connotations. When one gets aroused, the lips get fuller and redder. That is what red lipstick is designed to mimic.

Links Between Beauty and Fitness

Athletic abilities are correlated with attractiveness. Professor John Manning studied the link between attractiveness and athletic ability, and his research found that facial symmetry was the mediating factor in the correlation between beauty and athletic ability. The more symmetrical the face, the faster the runner. This observation might be explained by the advantage of better aerodynamics in more symmetrical athletes.

Similar research was conducted by Erik Postma, an evolutionary biologist at the University of Zurich. In his research, Postma investigated whether excelling at endurance sports is associated with physical attractiveness, and he also looked at whether more attractive people perform better as athletes. Postma was also curious to find out whether greater physical endurance makes athletes seem more appealing.

A study published in the journal *Biology Letters* posed the same questions. In this study, 80 participants were asked to rate the attractiveness of cyclists who competed in the 2012 Tour de France. Racers who placed in the top 10 percent of the race also scored 25 percent higher on looks than the racers who performed less well. In other words, there appears to be a strong connection between whom we find attractive and greater athletic endurance.

So, do the results of these studies mean that we are drawn to people with an endurance edge, like the top Tour de France racers? Do these results confirm theories of human evolution that have been popularized in the book *Born to Run?* Do these findings provide evidence to support evolutionary psychology theory that the survival of early humans strongly depended on their ability run long distances to escape predators and hunt down food? If so, having greater physical endurance would be a very appealing skill.

Perhaps, higher physical endurance can be detected in people's faces, which makes them more attractive? Postma was intrigued by his previous observations, so he conducted further research to elucidate the nature of the link between physical endurance and attractiveness. He requested 800 people to take an online survey that depicted 80 Tour de France racers' head-shots. The participants were requested to rate each photo on its attractiveness on a scale of 1 to 5, where a score of 1 was labelled "ugly" and a score of 5 was labelled "cue catcalls."

The research investigators ensured that participants remained ignorant to how each cyclist did in the race. The research found a significant positive correlation between attractiveness and race performance, but the reasons for these results were unclear. Did the cyclists who were rated higher in attractiveness have a greater air of confidence? A certain angle of cheekbone? Did they just look healthier and more fit? After performing numerous statistical tests in an attempt to elucidate the reasons for these results, Postma commented, "I was frankly skeptical that I would find something. I think I've done everything I could to disprove myself, but it seems very robust."

While there's a dearth of research on endurance athletes and attractiveness, there are studies that have investigated whether overall fitness is associated with greater attractiveness. One study found that women are more attracted to the faces of highly-rated NFL quarterbacks than quarterbacks whose performance is less highly rated.

Nevertheless, the results of these studies are not always so clear-cut. In another study, women were more drawn to the bodies of men who scored better on fitness tests, but the researchers observed no link between athletic ability and facial attractiveness. Postma noted that people readily accept that other species might have evolved with a preference for certain physical characteristics in a mate. Female elk, for example, are drawn to the males with the loudest call.

But when it comes to humans, it's a different story. Postma observed that people are more resistant to the idea that evolutionary priming plays a significant role in human attraction. He observed, "A lot of people tend to think that as humans we stand above; that we are not animals anymore."

So, it would seem overall that the research supports the idea that there are many biological influences on the human perception of outward beauty. The Golden Ratio provides some insight into what the human eye finds appealing, but there's much more to be understood in regards to what truly makes a person beautiful.

CHAPTER THREE

SPF Is Your BFF

One of the questions people ask me most frequently is "What is the cheapest and simplest way I can start taking charge of my beauty"? I never hesitate to say that it is sun protection. It has been proven that sun protection can prevent skin cancers, like basal cell carcinoma, squamous cell carcinoma, and malignant melanoma. In my years in dermatology, I have seen each one of these skin cancers numerous times, and in most cases, the patient regrets not wearing sunblock in previous years. If appropriate, I remind them that they were children and probably didn't know any better, and their parents probably weren't as educated about the effects of the sun as we are now. In truth, extensive knowledge about the benefits of sunblock is a relatively new development. Good sunblock protection can prevent skin cancer, but it can also prevent premature aging. Below is a picture of the face of a female truck driver whose left side was exposed to sun through an open window during her years of driving.

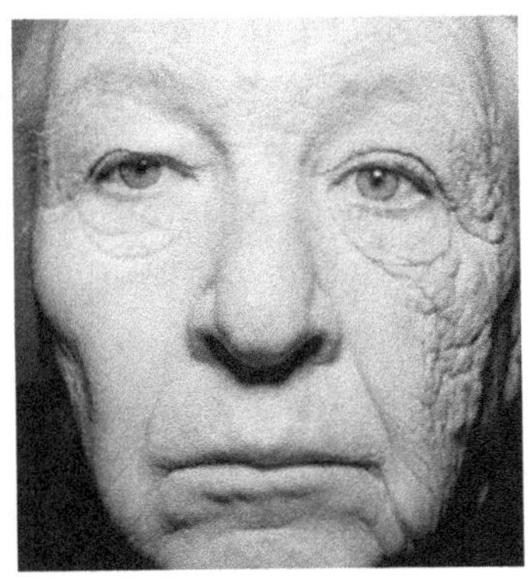

What Do You Look for in an SPF BFF?

When choosing sun protection products, you need to look at both the level of protection and the quality of the ingredients. What is SPF? SPF stands for "sun protection factor," and it is a measure of a sunscreen's ability to prevent UVB rays from damaging the skin. SPF refers to protection from only UVB rays (which cause sunburn), but not UVA rays, which are linked to deeper skin damage. There are currently no rating scales for UVA in the US. Both UVA and UVB rays contribute to the risk of skin cancer. Therefore, it is very important to look for a sunscreen that is broad-spectrum so that you know it will protect you from both UVA and UVB rays.

The number of the SPF indicates the length of time that your skin is protected from sunburn. Think of this rating as a measure of time it would take you to burn if you were not wearing sunscreen as opposed to the time it would take with sunscreen on. Which number you need may depend on your skin type. For example, if you are a person who starts getting sunburned within five minutes in the sun without any protection, applying sunscreen with an SPF of 30 would protect you for 30×5 minutes (or 150 minutes) before you begin to burn. Of course, there are several factors that could affect this, which will result in your needing more or less sunblock. The general guidelines is that you need to protect your skin between the hours of 10am and 3pm. Avoid being exposed to the sun during the highest peak of sun strength. If you reside in a part of the world where there is stronger sun penetration, like near the equator, then sun protection is particularly important. Wearing sun protective clothing might reduce your need for sunblock while reflective light from snow or water might increase your need for protection.

The American Academy of Dermatology recommends using sunscreen with an SPF of at least 30, which blocks 97 percent of the sun's UVB rays. Higher number SPFs block slightly more of the sun's UVB rays, but no sunscreen can block 100 percent of the sun's UVB rays. I tell my patients to choose their product based on an SPF of between 30 and 50, the quality of the ingredients (go with mineral/physical blockers like zinc and titanium), and the ease of reapplication. The difference in protection afforded by the SPF numbers is not proportionate. If you think that an SPF of 30 will be double the protection of SPF 15, you are mistaken. The difference is that SPF 15 blocks 93 percent of UVB rays while SPF 30 blocks 97 percent. As the SPF rating increases, the incremental increases in the percentage of sun protection are smaller.

What Does "Broad-Spectrum" Mean?

"Broad-spectrum" means that the product provides protection against both UVA and UVB ultraviolet rays. UV radiation that reaches the Earth from the sun has different wavelengths—some short, some long. These waves are classified as UVA, UVB, or UBC. UVA is the longest of the three, and UVB is the shorter wavelength. UVC is absorbed by the ozone layer and does not reach the earth.

Both UVA and UVB penetrate the atmosphere and play an important role in conditions like premature skin aging, eye damage, and skin cancers. Researchers believe ultraviolet radiation also suppresses the immune system, reducing your ability to fight skin cancers like basal cell carcinoma, squamous cell carcinoma, and melanoma.

What Are the Differences between UVA and UVB?

UVA has a longer wavelength than UVB, and it also accounts for 90 to 95 percent of the UV radiation that reaches the earth. UVB has a shorter wavelength, but it contains a higher energy of radiation. It makes up only about 5 to 10 percent of our solar radiation. UVB rays have high energy and can damage surface epidermal layers and cause sunburn. UVB is strongest between 10am and 4pm from April to October in the Northern Hemisphere. These waves do not penetrate glass, so they cannot affect you in your car or home.

UVA is present equally throughout the daylight hours and through all the seasons, and these rays can penetrate clouds and glass. It's important to use sun protection, even on overcast days during the fall, spring, and winter, and also while in the car. UVA penetrates deeper layers of skin and causes tanning. Tanning is your body's natural reaction to injury to the skin and the skin's DNA.

However, both types of UV rays can cause skin cancer because they damage skin cells and alter the DNA. Both UVA and UVB rays also contribute to premature aging of the skin. This is why a broad-spectrum sunblock is important to protect you from both UVA and UVB damage.

UV Radiation and the Skin

     Take Charge of Your Beauty

What Is in Your Sunscreen?

There are two different types of sunscreen ingredients: physical (also known as mineral) and chemical. Both use different mechanisms for protecting skin and maintaining stability in sunlight. Think of the two types like this: chemical sunscreens act like a sponge while the physical sunscreens act like a wall. The words "sunscreen" and "sunblock" are often used interchangeably. "Sunscreens" refer to products that screen the UV rays, like chemical ingredients that absorb them. "Sunblock" does as it states, and it often achieves this with mineral/physical blockers.

Physical sunblock contains particles that reflect the sun's rays away from the skin. They don't get absorbed into the skin as chemical sunscreens do. They also do not react by releasing any potential harmful by-products and can be washed off easily. The most common negative comment I hear about physical sunscreen is that these products tend to leave white streaks on your skin and may be a little thicker, so it may take a little longer to apply and wash off. However, higher-end products made with these ingredients have minimized these problems.

Two ingredients approved by the FDA for use as physical sunscreens are titanium dioxide and zinc oxide. Both of these minerals offer protection against both UVA and UVB damage. Mineral or physical blockers are considered safe and FDA-approved. Titanium dioxide protects against UVB rays, but not the full spectrum of UVA rays. Zinc oxide protects against the entire spectrum of UVB and UVA rays.

Chemical sunscreens form a thin layer on top of the skin and absorb UV rays before they reach the skin. Because it is absorbed into the skin, chemical sunscreen can lead to skin irritation and other adverse reactions. Plus, the ingredients can generate cell-damaging free radicals when exposed to the sun.

Ingredients Commonly Found in Chemical Sunscreens

In addition to sunscreen-related skin allergies and irritants, some chemical UV filters have been said to mimic hormones. I will now discuss the major issues with the most commonly-used chemicals.

Avobenzone

Avobenzone is one of the most common UVA chemical filters in sunscreen ingredients, and it is very unstable and degrades in sunlight. It is considered to be one of the best protectors from UVA rays and is considered safe. It does have a tendency to degrade significantly in light, lessening its sun protection capabilities. For this reason, most sunscreens containing this ingredient also include photo-stabilizing ingredients, like octocrylene, but this is also an irritant.

Octinoxate

Octinoxate is one of the most common ingredients found in sunscreens with SPF. It helps other ingredients to be absorbed more readily. While allergic reactions from octinoxate aren't common, hormone disruption is: The chemical's effects on estrogen can be harmful for humans and wildlife. This can happen when it dissolves in water. Though SPF products are designed to protect skin from sun-induced aging, octinoxate may actually be a culprit for premature aging since it produces free radicals that can damage skin.

Octisalate is an organic compound used as an ingredient in sunscreens and cosmetics to absorb the full range of UVB rays from the sun. It is a colorless liquid with an oily consistency that often emits a mildly floral fragrance. It has been approved for use in concentrations of up to 5 percent.

Octocrylene

When this chemical is exposed to UV light, it absorbs the rays and produces oxygen radicals that can damage cells and cause mutations. It is readily absorbed and may accumulate within the body in measurable amounts. Plus, it can be toxic to the environment.

Oxybenzone

Oxybenzone is a chemical that can cause an eczema-like allergic reaction, which can spread beyond the exposed area and last long after you're out of the sun. Experts also suspect that oxybenzone disrupts hormones (i.e., mimics, blocks, and alters hormone levels), which can disrupt your endocrine system. This additive warrants further study.

Potentially Harmful Ingredients

Retinyl Palmitate

Retinyl palmitate is a combination of retinol (vitamin A) and palmitic acid, an ingredient found in tropical plants, like palm and coconut, and it could be potentially damaging. When exposed to the sun's UV rays, retinol compounds break down and produce destructive free radicals that are toxic to cells, damage DNA, and may lead to cancer. In fact, FDA studies have shown that retinyl palmitate may speed the development of malignant cells and skin tumors when applied to skin before sun exposure, so steer clear of skin sun products with this ingredient.

Homosalate

Once this ingredient has been absorbed, homosalate accumulates in our bodies faster than we can get rid of it, which becomes toxic and disrupts our hormones.

Paraben Preservatives

Associated with both acute and chronic side effects, parabens induce allergic reactions, hormone disruption, and they have been linked with developmental and reproductive toxicity. It is suspected that parabens and other chemicals in underarm cosmetics may contribute to the rising incidence of breast cancer.

These chemical blockers have pros and cons. The most common perceived difficulty is that they are known to be more irritating for sensitive skin. Have you ever felt stinging in your eyes after applying sunscreen? It very likely resulted from a chemical blocker. Nevertheless, stinging is hardly the worst effect considering that there is evidence to suggest that it is toxic and possibly carcinogenic.

How Can You Choose the Best Product?

There are many safe sunscreens and sunblocks on the market now due to the public's demand for safer and more effective products. Health food and natural grocery stores stock quite a few. The Environmental Working Group has a guide to sunscreens that recommends specific products for specific uses.

Water Resistant versus Waterproof?

Now that you are learning the importance of sunblock and identifying the best product for you, it is also important to learn how to protect yourself from the sun when sweating or in the water. Water -resistant formulas stand up to water better than regular sunscreens, offering protection for 40 minutes, and waterproof sunscreens are formulated to last twice as long (80 minutes) as water-resistant formulas.

How is the length of time for protection determined? The tests are conducted in independent labs with human subjects. The sunscreen is applied to a person's arm, which is then submerged in a jacuzzi. If, after the submersion in hot water, the sunscreen still protects to the same degree as the SPF written on the label, then the sunscreen can make a water-resistant or waterproof claim.

Sprays

Sunscreen sprays are very popular, but there is concern that they may be an inhalation risk and may not provide a thick and even coating on the skin. The FDA has asked companies that manufacture sprays to supply more data to prove that spray sunscreens protect skin and pose no safety hazard, so watch for changes in the regulation of these products.

I personally avoid any aerosol sprays. If using a spray, apply it in your hands and then rub it to the area you want to apply it to. Do not spray it directly to the face since you want to avoid inhaling the sunscreen and its ingredients. Avoid using sprays indoors or in non-ventilated areas. I would like add that I do recommend sun protection sprays for the scalp. Many of the hats people wear outdoors don't offer enough protection for the head.

What Is Your Skin Type?

The Fitzpatrick Scale

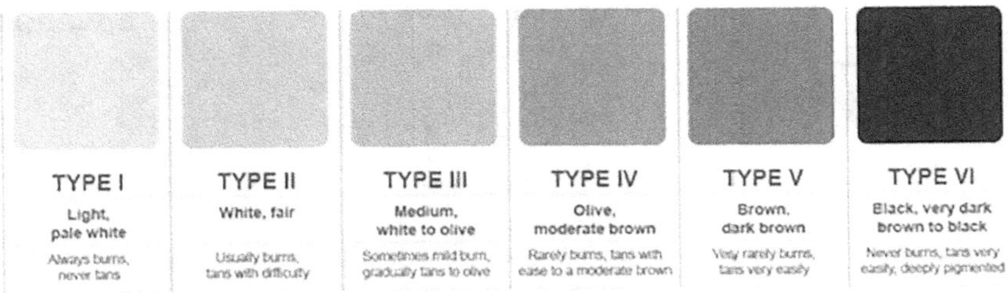

The Fitzpatrick scale is a classification of human skin color. It was developed in 1975 by Dr. Thomas Fitzpatrick as a way to estimate the response of different skin types to ultraviolet light. Below is the chart with the Fitzpatrick scale of type one through type six:

It is a misconception that people with darker skin do not need sunscreen. Skin types 4 to 6 are my patients who say, "Oh, I never burn." Having darker skin can produce a false sense of confidence. Anyone can get skin cancer, regardless of race or color. While darker skin produces more of the pigment called melanin, which does help to protect the skin, it doesn't provide complete protection.

It is believed that a type five or six requires an SPF protection of only 15. This is still not enough protection, and these patients need to concern themselves with sunscreen and reapplication as well. The ultraviolet rays still have the potential to damage skin and lead to often undiagnosed skin cancer, and they can cause hyper-pigmentation and premature aging as well.

Due to some of these misconceptions, darker skinned patients tend to have skin cancer screenings less frequently than light skinned people. Unfortunately, due to this, when dark skinned people have a skin cancer, it is often diagnosed in the late stages. This can be very dangerous with malignant melanoma. People with darker skin are more susceptible to a very dangerous form of melanoma, called acral lentiginous melanoma; it typically appears on the palms of the hands and soles of the feet. The famous Jamaican singer and musician, Bob Marley, died of this type of melanoma when he was only 36 years old.

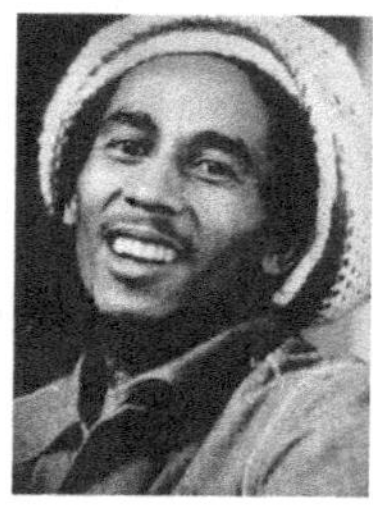

Skin Checks

The American Academy of Dermatology recommends that all people have skin checks annually. Thorough skin examinations should include the scalp, hands, feet, and toes. It is also recommended that patients self-monitor between their annual visits. I advise my patients that if there's any change between appointments to come in and have it checked by a medical skin professional, like a dermatologist or a physician assistant/nurse practitioner who specializes in dermatology.

The medical providers who specialize in dermatology have many years of experience with patients, and they have the training to differentiate between benign and suspicious-looking lesions. In many offices, they also utilize equipment, like a microscope, to aid them in their decisions.

When conducting self-monitoring, it is useful to remember the ABCDE chart of melanoma. This describes the types of changes in moles that may be dangerous and that warrant an exam from a professional.

Additionally, certain skin cancers are caused by factors other than UV rays. Other factors to consider are genetics and environmental influences, like tanning booths.

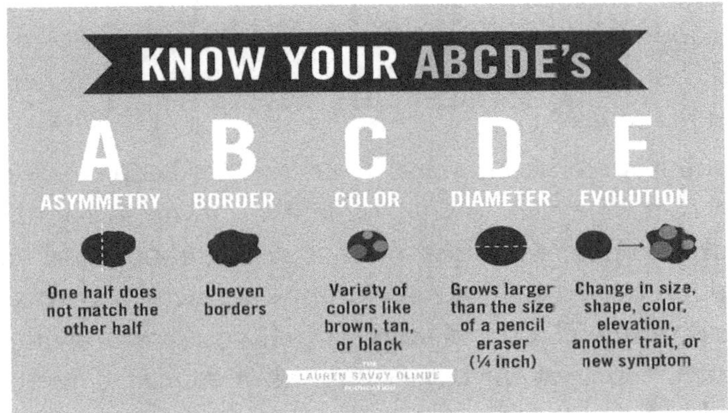

Why Are Tanning Beds So Dangerous?

Up to 90 percent of melanomas are estimated to be caused by ultraviolet exposure. This includes UV exposure from the sun and from artificial sources, like tanning beds. The World Health Organization's international agency of research on cancer has classified tanning beds and tanning (sun) lamps in the very highest cancer-risk category. They state that tanning beds are carcinogenic to humans and are in the same category as hazardous substances, like plutonium.

Unfortunately, the tanning industry has led consumers to believe that a short exposure in the tanning booths can help with vitamin D deficiencies and produce a less harmful "natural tan" due to a short exposure time in a booth. The truth is that the majority of tanning booths use UVA radiation, and UVB radiation is needed for the body to produce vitamin D. The fact is, all necessary vitamin D can be found in a healthy diet or a vitamin supplement. If you are truly concerned about your vitamin D levels, consult your doctor to have your level measured, not a tanning salon!

The connection between UV radiation and melanoma is clear. However, the popularity of tanning booths is greater than ever. Researchers believe that there is an addictive component to tanning. UV light has been shown to increase the release of endorphins—the feel-good chemicals that relieve pain and generate feelings of well-being. It is believed that this is potentially what leads to an addiction to tanning.

Tanning is an indication that your skin has been exposed to UV radiation, so it is never known to be safe. Contrary to popular belief, it is possible to get a sunburn in any tanning booth, and your eyes are also at increased risk of developing cataracts or corneal burns. The FDA and the CDC both suggest that you avoid using tanning beds in order to prevent developing skin cancer. There really is no such thing as safety in a tanning bed. Aside from the risk of developing skin cancer, exposure to UV rays causes your skin to age prematurely, and it also adversely affects your immune system

So now you know that the greatest cosmetic gift you can give yourself takes only commitment, awareness, and a trip to the local store. No surgery or professionals are needed! I truly hope that the information in this chapter motivates you to take the next step towards giving yourself this gift.

Take Charge of Your Beauty

CHAPTER FOUR

Saving Face, One Wrinkle at a Time

The explosion of aesthetic treatments can all be attributed to the introduction of the Botox® cosmetic. Although Botox® became a household name in the early 2000s, the benefits and effects of the bacterium have been well known and widely studied since the 1800s. For my history buff beauties, here is a brief review on botulinum bacterium.

This "wrinkle eraser" has a colorful history, and I love to say it took a village (and close to a century of scientists and physicians studying the bacterium) to create a safe product for therapeutic use. The name "Botox" is the patented name of a drug made from the toxins produced by the bacterium, botulinum bacterium.

The bacterium was first documented in 1817 by a German physician, named Justinus Kerner, who was the first to find a possible therapeutic use for this newly discovered toxin, which he called "sausage poison"; the toxin was thus named because patients who ate contaminated sausages developed a unique group of symptoms that resembled symptoms brought about by bacterium botulinum. In particular, Dr. Kerner noted that the poison paralyzed muscles. At this point, he began to speculate that this substance had a possible application in therapy for certain medical conditions. Kerner also observed that botulism patients experienced dry mouth and eyes, and he suggested that the toxin might be used to control excessive sweating, which led the FDA to approve its use for hyperhidrosis.

It wasn't until 1897 that microbiologist Emile Pierre van Ermengen identified and named the bacterium, Clostridium botulinum, although we will refer to it by its other name, botulinum bacterium. Research on this substance continued sporadically until a discovery led to a possible application for therapeutic treatment. In the 1950s, Arnold Burgen and Vernon Brooks from McGill University discovered that the botulism toxin works by blocking the release of acetylcholine (a type of neurotransmitter) from motor nerve terminals. This meant that the toxin would be useful for calming hyperactive muscles.

In the early 1970s, Edward Schantz showed that injecting minute amounts of the botulinum toxin into the hind legs of chicks caused local denervation. Around this time, an ophthalmologist from San Francisco, Dr. Alan Scott, was looking for a treatment for his patients who suffered from strabismus (crossed eyes). Dr. Scott and Dr. Schantz found that injecting minute amounts of botulinum into the muscles around the eyes of monkeys with strabismus produced a long-lasting correction, and without any systemic effects. These observations by Dr. Scott led to the first clinical trial in 1977 for humans with strabismus. In this research, a minute amount of botulinum was injected into the muscles around the eyes. Dr. Scott's manufactured product was originally named Oculinum and was later licensed and acquired by Allergan, who still manufactures Botox today.

Within a few years, the FDA approved Botox for strabismus, blepharospasm (involuntary, repetitive movement of the muscles surrounding the eyes), and cervical dystonia (involuntary contractions of the neck and shoulder muscles resulting in head tilting and moderate to severe pain).

By the late 1980s, over 10,000 patients had received Botox for strabismus. An ophthalmologist from Vancouver, Canada, Dr. Jean Carruthers, noticed an unexpected result in a patient's brow and expression line between the eyebrows, which produced a more relaxed and youthful appearance after injection. Dr. Jean Carruthers shared this observation with her husband, dermatologist, Dr. Alastair Carruthers. As a dermatologist, patients often asked him about reducing wrinkles. This casual dinner conversation led them to conduct their own studies on patients.

As good news spread about the wrinkle-reducing properties of Botox between 1992 and 1997, its popularity grew so rapidly that Allergan's supply temporarily ran out! By 2000, the FDA approved Botox for injection into wrinkles in the area between the brows.

Botox is currently being studied as a possible application in juvenile cerebral palsy.

History of Approved Indications for Botox in the United States and Europe

1989	Strabismus and Blepharospasm
2000	Cervical Dystonia
2002	Glabellar (frown lines)
2004	Axillary Hyperhidrosis (excessive sweating under the arms)
2010	Upper limb spasticity and chronic migraine
2011	Overactive bladder
2013	Crow's feet and wrinkle indication
2014	Lower limb spasticity

Is Botox Safe?

Most people's concerns about the safety of the Botox toxin are usually resolved when they learn about the history of botulinum toxin. I often discuss this with patients who are slightly fearful of any potential side effects when they are interested in getting rid of their wrinkles. I always remind patients that there are more FDA approved indications of Botox for medical conditions than there are for cosmetic use. These medical conditions have been treated with Botox for longer and with greater frequently than Botox has been used in aesthetics.

Neuromodulator What? Neurotoxin What?

We often refer to the botulism toxin as Botox, but the technically correct way to refer to it is as a neuromodulator. The reason why this terminology has been changed is that Botox is a branded name. Allergan owns this product and has trademarked their specific strain of the botulinum toxin, Botox®. It was the first neuromodulator approved in the United States. Botox® remains the most commonly used name throughout the world for this neuromodulator. In the United States, there are three FDA approved neuromodulators for aesthetic purposes: 1) Botox, 2) Dysport, and 3) Xeomin.

The differences among these three products have been argued among injectors and patients. Botox was the first to become available and continues to dominate the cosmetic market in the United States; it also has the most FDA-approved indications. Dysport and Xeomin have several of the same FDA-approved indications and are often used (off-label) similarly to Botox. Many of the perceived differences among these three products are reflected by the subjective experiences of the injector or the patient in terms of their experiences and results. Their molecular weight may vary slightly, but their purpose and mechanism of action are the same in all three.

Resistance to Botox?

Therapeutic failure or disappointment in Botox for cosmetic use is very uncommon and has only been reported in a few instances. It is believed that resistance to treatment is due to the production of antibodies to the neurotoxin. Antibody development is highly complex and not yet fully understood, but it is believed to be determined by the immune system of the patient. The cumulative dose does not seem to be as important as the individual patient's immune reaction. Patients who are treated with high doses, such as 300 units of Botox or higher (which is never done in one session of an aesthetic procedure), and at frequent intervals seem the most likely to develop antibodies.

Cosmetic patients who are treated with Botox typically receive 25 to 75 units at intervals of several months, and are extremely unlikely to develop resistance. According to Allergan, only 1 to 2 percent of patients develop antibodies to Botox, and the correlation between these antibodies and failed clinical response is not clear. Therapeutic failure due to antibodies has been reported for both Dysport and Botox, while none has been reported for Xeomin. Fortunately, all currently used products have similar efficacy, safety profiles, and mechanisms of action, but the role of complex proteins in antibody development is still under investigation.

Common Botox Questions

Do I need Botox?

Needing and wanting are two different things. I am yet to meet a patient who wouldn't love to be without wrinkles. If you are investigating the possibility of smoothing out your existing lines and preventing new ones, then Botox would be the right choice for you! This injection is designed to relax muscles and reduce lines and wrinkles on your face. It is commonly injected to treat frown lines, forehead creases, crows feet, upper lip lines, and lines on the lower face and neck areas. Botox use for the prevention of wrinkles has increased in the recent years.

How do I choose a Botox provider?

1. Referrals

    Referrals are always the best way to find someone you trust! Ask a friend who has had the treatment done regularly and find out where they go.

2. Check Manufacturers' Websites

    It is crucial that you confirm whether your injector is treating you with a quality product. All three companies that make neurotoxins, including Allergan (Botox), Galderma (Dysport), and Merz (Xeomin), list site-approved providers of their products.

3. Credentials

    Nowadays, Botox can be found everywhere! Primary care physicians, obstetricians, gynecologists, dentists, and medical spas in the mall (and even pediatricians!) are now offering the treatment. Botox injections may not be a complex procedure like a surgery, but a sound knowledge of the human anatomy, muscles, and how muscles work together is absolutely critical.

    When Botox was first introduced for cosmetic purposes, it was offered only by dermatologists, ophthalmologists, or plastic surgeons. However, these days, some of the country's best injectors are nurses and physician assistants. While the medical specialists are often busy with surgeries, the mid-level providers have gathered many years of training and expertise. Botox (or any other neuromodulator) is not as simple as injecting it into the face. It takes skill and technique to get good, natural results.

    Look for a provider who has been practicing this specialization for several years. These providers will often have an established location and reputation. Avoid getting treated by someone who is doing it on the side and/or at someone's home. How would you contact them if there is an issue? How do you know whether their products are quality products? A static location and a reputable injector are likely indications that you will receive the best quality product.

An established and respectable provider cannot afford to give you anything but the best! They want you to be a long-term, happy, and beautiful patient. Pick someone who has numerous, solid reviews over someone who offers a discount. Often discounts are offered by people who are learning and people with poor technique. Unsightly results from a bad injection can last 3 to 4 months. Although you can cannot trust everything you read on review pages, if the practitioner was negligent, it would reflect in their reviews.

4. Good Consultation: Go with Your Gut!

A good consultation will tell you a lot about a practice and the provider. The provider should seek to gather a thorough medical history, which they should document throughout the course of the consultation. Botox is a medical procedure, so the practitioner needs to assess whether you are a safe candidate for the treatment. Remember, even though Botox is a household name, it is still a medical procedure. Check your state and see who can legally perform the procedure.

Here in California, the injector must be a licensed physician assistant (PA), nurse practitioner (NP), or physician before being seen by a registered nurse (RN). Botox is considered a prescription, so a patient must be evaluated and cleared as a candidate before being injected by a PA, NP, or physician.

The consultation should ease all of your concerns, and your provider should be confident and happy to answer all of your questions. Access to the provider's before-and-after pictures should also ease any hesitation.

Another last and important side note to think about during your consultation is to look at WHO is injecting you. Do they share the same aesthetic beliefs? Are they over-injected? People tend to vary in how they view beauty and aesthetics. If your provider is over-filled, you might end up looking the same! If you still need reassurance, Allergan, Mertz, and Galderma can all be contacted by telephone; you can then confirm whether your office location has an active account.

5. Global Assessment

My global assessment includes my overall impressions online, my staff interaction, and ultimately, how confident I feel with an injector. I never recommend basing any of your decisions on cost. You only have one face, but Botox effects (the good ones and the complications) can last for four months. Therefore, it is better to get a qualified and experienced injector.

Does Botox hurt?

I often get asked this question, and I think to myself, "Not as much as aging." Botox injections require a very small needle. The needles are so small and quick, that at the most, it feels like a small pinch. To avoid any discomfort, some people may offer topical numbing cream. I rarely find topical numbing cream necessary. We utilize ice packs just moments before injection to take the edge off. For our female patients, I always recommend avoiding any cosmetic procedure either a week before or during your period because women tend to be more sensitive to pain during this time.

Are there any side effects of Botox?

Every drug has side effects, and Botox is no exception. Luckily, the side effects of Botox tend to be minor and short-lived. In one to five percent of cases, there can be mild droopiness of the eyelid or eyebrow, which usually goes away within two weeks, and some patients experience slight bruising. This is more common in patients that may present with minor facial drooping, or it can also happen with slight injector mishaps. Some anatomical variances can also make a patient more susceptible to brow drooping. Brow drop or eyelid drop, although very uncommon, can happen with the best of injectors.

Advanced injectors understand areas to avoid to prevent brow or eyelid drop, but the size of a person's forehead or over dilution (which means product can spread towards undesired muscles nearby), poor technique, or unique anatomy (e.g., patient could have had scar tissue or previous surgery unknown to the injector, which can affect movement) can cause these side effects.

Another possible side effect is bruising. Bruising is not common, but it can occur and is more often around the crow's feet. Less than 3 percent of patients may experience eyelid swelling, discomfort, or pain at the injection sites, or headaches and temporary eye problems, like blurry vision, double vision, or dry eyes.

How many injections will I receive?

The amount of injections required depends on the areas where you want to receive it. Certain areas, like the forehead and neck, can significantly vary, depending on the size of the area and the number and depth of neck lines. So many times after telling my patients how many units I recommend, I get looks of horror! When I ask my patients why, they invariably respond that they think 50 units equals 50 shots! The table below depicts the average amount of injections that I recommend per area. Remember, injections do not equal units!

Average Number of Recommended Botox Injections

Glabellar (between brows)	5
Forehead	3-8 (Depends on size of forehead, and some advanced injectors do mini micro injections)
Crows feet	2-4 per side (average 3)
Bunny lines	2 (one on each side of the nasal bridge)
Chin	2-3
Masseters	3
Upper lip	2-4

How much does Botox cost?

Botox can be charged per area (glabellar, forehead, crow's feet, upper lip, chin, masseter), or per unit. In most offices, including ours, practitioners charge per unit. Since Botox is not a cookie-cutter treatment, we believe that the price should only reflect the specific amount of muscle contractions required for your area of treatment. Nationwide, the price per unit may vary between $10–20 per unit. The toxins arrive dehydrated and must be reconstituted, so some doctors either over-dilute or under-dilute. The quality of the result always depends on who is on the other end of the needle!

How many units will I need?

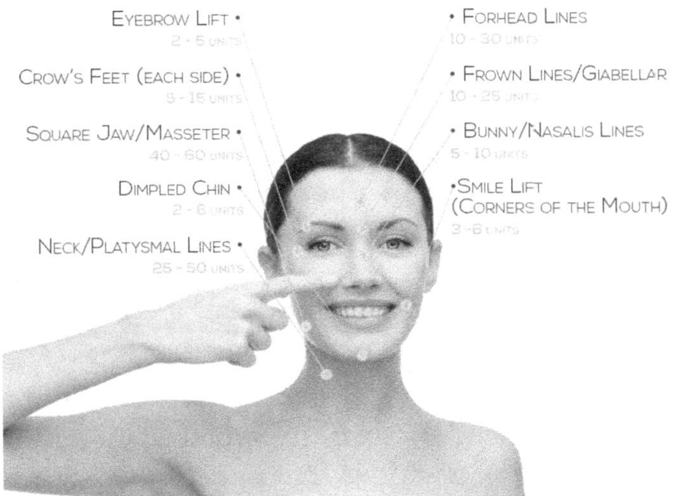

How long does the treatment take?

After the consultation, the actual treatment takes less than 10 minutes.

How long until I see results?

It takes a few days for neuromodulators to take effect. The effects may be first noticed in 72 hours but can take up to 7–10 days. You might be asked to return after your first treatment so that your provider can assess your response. The first set of injections might only yield partial results. This is most likely because your provider wants to start with a conservative and natural approach to gauge how you will respond to the treatment. For patients with established lines that are visible without animation (i.e., facial movement), it might take a couple of treatments to train your muscles to relax. I do not recommend adding more neuromodulators until at least 10 days after the initial injection.

What happens if I still have a deep crease after 10 days of my first treatment?

Always communicate any concerns with your injector. I personally feel that it is an honor for you to trust me with your face, so if it's not perfect, tell them. After years of repeating the same facial expressions, expression lines will eventually form in these areas, even when you are not pulling the facial expression that caused the lines. The only way to help prevent these lines from appearing at rest is to apply Botox to the muscles that are used to form the expression, which will soften their movement.

However, there are many factors that contribute to the results of your Botox treatment. When treating patients with Botox, the goal is not to erase all of their lines, but rather, to create a naturally smoother appearance. Your treatment result depends on how much Botox is used, its placement (which muscles are injected as well as the location of the wrinkles within the muscles), the strength of the muscles treated, and the technique and expertise of your injector.

If you still have a deep crease, your injector's first observation should be on the results of relaxing those muscles. If the patient still has movement in the area, then it is recommended to add more Botox to the area to completely relax those muscles that contribute to the crease. If the patient attempts to constrict the muscle and they have no movement at all, then no further Botox should be added because the Botox has done its job in relaxing the muscles.

Botox is not capable of filling in lines because it is not a dermal filler, so it makes sense that your lines will not disappear with Botox alone. The frown area between the eyebrows is a common area for a combination treatment of Botox (to quieten the facial expression) and a dermal filler, such as Restylane or Juvederm, to lift the line and create a smoother appearance.

How long do my results last?

On average, you can expect to repeat the treatment every three to four months to maintain your results. After repeated treatments at this interval, many patients will eventually notice a longer-term effect as the muscles remain quiet over a longer period and require fewer treatments to suppress their activity.

With a thorough understanding of the clinical research and history of botulinum toxin, it is easy to feel confident in its use. Botox is now the most common cosmetic procedure performed in the world. Although it has achieved its popularity in cosmetics, it is still used in far greater quantities worldwide for treating medical conditions. It cannot be refuted that Botox cosmetic is the leader of all anti-aging tools. It has also been found to be a leading treatment in the prevention of the early signs of aging.

Linda Rank

Take Charge of Your Beauty

CHAPTER FIVE

Enhance & Restore—How Dermal Fillers Can Help Maintain Your Natural Volume

Some of the most frequent comments I hear from my clients are "I want to look my best," "My face has dropped, and I have lines that I swear weren't there until recently," and "I look so tired, even after 8 hours of sleep, regular exercise, and a great diet." T hese comments are often followed up with comments like "What can I do to fix this?"

In chapter One, I discussed intrinsic and extrinsic aging. As we age, we lose collagen and elastin, which leads to loss of volume and our skin becoming more wrinkled, etc. To explain how these problems can be treated, you first need to understand what collagen and elastin are and what they do for us.

The simplest explanation is that collagen is responsible for volume. You can think of it as the structure and framework of the skin, which gives the skin its strength and foundation. Elastin is what gives the skin its "snap back." Its function is to return the skin to its original state of origin after the skin is stretched or contracted. It can be thought of as like a rubber band because it snaps back.

Collagen and elastin work synergistically, and they are responsible for the youthful, taut look of our skin during adolescence and during our twenties. As with most things in the human body, as we get older, we produce less of these two vital proteins.

If you are reading this book it is likely that you have already started to notice that your skin does not snap back as well as it did in the past, and unfortunately, the tell-tale signs are often sagging around your eyes, mouth, jaw line, and neck.

As part of the skin assessment process, some medical practices are able to tell you how much collagen and elastin you have in your skin prior to any treatments or procedures.

So, what can be done to restore the skin's thickness and snap back? To help answer that question, I will discuss dermal fillers and how they can help maintain, restore, and enhance the appearance of your skin. The most obvious questions are:

- What are they and what do they do?
- How can dermal fillers help with the aging process?
- How can fillers help to restore and even enhance the appearance of your skin?

What Are Dermal Fillers?

Dermal fillers are a cosmetic medicine. They are products made mostly from a combination of natural and synthetic materials . Facial fillers are FDA-approved prescription products, like collagen, hyaluronic acid, and calcium hydroxyl apatite, all of which are designed to improve the appearance of the skin via reducing the appearance of wrinkles, treating volume loss, and enhancing the appearance of the lips.

Facial fillers can be either temporary or longer-term treatments that are administered through a few small facial injections on specific areas of the face. There are a variety of fillers available, and each of these products is designed for different purposes, such as fine wrinkle reduction, adding volume, and lip augmentation. Facial fillers are designed to volumize creases and folds in the face in areas that have lost fat and collagen.

As noted in chapter One, dermal fillers are a non-invasive treatment, and they are also a mild and safe anti-aging treatment that provides long-lasting skin renewal to restore and enhances your skin. How long it lasts depends on the product, which area has been treated, and how your skin type responds to the treatment. In general, the deeper it is injected and the denser the filler, the greater its longevity.

How Do Dermal Fillers Help with the Aging Process?

Dermal fillers produce modest results, so for those of us who do not want to appear as if we have had work done, dermal fillers can be a great option. There are a lot of reasons why both men and women choose to get dermal fillers. You might notice that you have gradually lost volume in your face, such as your cheeks, which may have caused your face to lose some of its natural shape and definition. For example, your skin might feel loose or saggy, you might notice that you have new wrinkles, your existing lines might be getting deeper, or you might simply think that you are looking tired or older.

As mentioned briefly in chapter One, as we age, the skin will inevitably lose volume and elasticity because of decreases in collagen, elastin, and hyaluronic acid. Naturally, this causes a change in our facial contours, and it can lead us to feel that we look more tired and appear older than we feel.

There are a lot of reasons to consider dermal fillers that restore and enhance your skin and which also correct the visible signs of aging. As mentioned at the start of the book, we are remaining in the workforce for a lot longer than the generations before us. Having procedures done that help restore and enhance our looks may well help you to secure a new job, help you with sales, and most importantly, enhance your confidence in the workforce.

Fillers can restore and enhance in many ways that surpass even the very best skincare products. I am not suggesting of course that an excellent skincare regimen will not make a substantial difference in the appearance of your skin, but intrinsic and extrinsic factors of aging will eventually take their toll on your skin. Also, keep in mind that once you have had the treatments, excellent, well-formulated skincare products and sun protection will help keep your skin looking younger and healthier for longer!

How Do Dermal Fillers Work?

Dermal fillers are used to fill in and plump the skin as well as add volume. They produce a subtle effect that looks completely natural, and they are generally administered via small injections, with minimal discomfort and downtime. As a rule, the results are instantaneous, and an added benefit is that they help to keep your skin hydrated by attracting and holding water. In addition, they supplement the collagen and elastin of your skin, which improves the skin's structure and elasticity.

Types of Fillers and Their Usesr

Products listed below are common products currently used in the US. This will be an ongoing changing field.

Hyaluronic Acid Fillers

We all have hyaluronic acid (HA) in our skin, which has a key role in maintaining moisture in the skin, and our bodies also produce an enzyme called hyaluronidase that helps to degrade damaged or old HA. This is a continual, ongoing process in our skin and increases with some types of injuries to the skin. As we get older, this process slows down, which contributes to the visible signs of aging.

The dominant filler that is currently used by skin specialists is hyaluronic acid (HA), which is a synthetically produced product that can be injected directly into the skin. There are numerous types of HA fillers, and each of these fillers has different properties and uses. These differing physical properties determine where the product should be injected for best results, as well as how much should be injected.

Hyaluronic acid fillers come in varying levels of thickness, and so they are a flexible option to improve different sections of the face. Thinner HA fillers are more suitable for wrinkles, fine lines, and lips while thicker fillers are more suitable for deep wrinkles and volume loss.

Commonly-Used HA Fillers

Juvederm

Juvederm is a group of products that are made of a hyaluronic acid gel, which is designed to temporarily plump moderate to severe facial wrinkles and folds. Juvederm Voluma is a thicker HA dermal filler, and as such, it is a better option for achieving volume and contour in the cheeks because it is a more cohesive product. Juvederm Ultra Plus is a less cohesive product that is designed to plump and polish, so it is a better option for lines and shadows on the lower part of the face.

Juvederm Vollure is a product that uses a technology called Vycross to hold the hyaluronic acid together in a cohesive gel, which functions to keep the gel intact after it's injected into the skin. This technology links both high and low molecular weight hyaluronic acid while Juvederm's other products use Hylacross technology, which works via various degrees of crosslinking mainly high molecular weight hyaluronic acid to achieve a malleable gel that flows easily into the skin and creates a smooth natural look and feel.

The mixture of high and low hyaluronic acid in the Vycross technology creates a more connected gel, which can be molded to lift sunken skin. Juvederm Volbella is another HA filler that has been specifically developed for the lips and mouth area. The gel works by filling in lip lines and wrinkles, and the hyaluronic acid within attracts and retains moisture.

Although HA fillers are often a safer option, some HA products can result in blue discoloration of the skin, particularly in patients who have very fair skin.

Restylane and Belotero

Restylane is a biodegradable gel that is also made up of hyaluronic acid, and it is a soft tissue dermal filler that adds volume to the skin through small injections. It is designed to smooth facial folds and wrinkles around the mouth and eyes. Belotero is another HA filler that is better suited to treat superficial or fine lines, whereas other hyaluronic acid fillers may result in a less natural appearance. Belotero is intended for treatment areas, such as forehead wrinkles, frown lines, crow's feet, and smile or laugh lines.

A Brief Word on Viscosity and Particle Size of Hyaluronic Acid Fillers

Appropriate product selection is important for achieving optimal results with dermal fillers. Larger particle size or more viscous fillers achieve better results when they are injected deeply in the dermis while smaller particle size fillers or those with less viscosity are better suited for the treatment of superficial lines.

The newer dermal fillers use a technology called crosslinking, which is a composite dermal filler that is thought to increase longevity. Also, particle sizes differ between the different types of fillers. For example, the hyaluronic acid particles in Restylane are uniformly shaped while the HA particles in Juvederm are randomly shaped, and this variability in particle size is believed to be the reason for Juvederm's smooth gel-like consistency.

Additionally, Juvederm has thinner (Ultra) and thicker (Ultra Plus) versions, which means that these products were designed for different purposes. The greater particle size and slight crosslinking in Juverderm Ultra Plus compared with Juvederm Ultra means that Juverderm Ultra Plus is designated for deeper injections, which renders it more suitable for volumizing and contouring while Juverderm Ultra is better for more superficial lines.

Non-Hyaluronic Acid Fillers

There are other non-HA fillers that are widely used in the US, and among these fillers are Radiesse Radiesse and SculptraScupltra. Both these products contain long-lasting ingredients although Radiesse does have some limitations. Radiesse is typically used for deeper folds and furrows, but in combination with HA fillers for finer lines. Sculptra is a product that stimulates the production of collagen although it often requires multiple sessions of injections, and also, the results can take longer to appear while the body produces more of its own collagen.

Full facial rejuvenation is sometimes accomplished using Sculptra combined with HA fillers, and optimal results with skilled skin specialists can be achieved after several months. Radiesse is white in color and can sometimes show through the skin while Sculptra does not cause any discoloration.

Bellafill Bellafill is a combination of microsphere-enhanced bovine collagen and a local anesthetic . Bellafill is an FDA-approved dermal filler for permanent implantation into the skin for the correction of nasolabial folds (smile lines). It can be used in both women and men. Bellafill is a non-absorbable dermal filler, unlike many other dermal fillers that are absorbed and require re-injection. Bellafill is also used for moderate to severe acne scars on the cheeks.

Which Type of Injectable Dermal Filler Treatment Is Best for You?

I really want to emphasize that the technique and experience of injectors make a substantial difference to the results that you can expect. The technique and experience of the skin specialist can also impact how many syringes of filler are needed to achieve the best results. Fillers are a more difficult treatment than Botox, so it is critical that you carefully research your skincare specialist's experience and read their reviews before you make a commitment.

The right type of injectable dermal filler treatment to achieve a patient's goals for improvements in the appearance of the face can be determined by the following factors:

Area of the Face: Some fillers are better suited than others for certain areas of the face due to properties of the filler (such as the dermal filler's thickness) and the area that is being treated.

Depth of Creases and Facial Wrinkles: Typically, thicker fillers are more effective at treating deep folds and wrinkles while lighter fillers tend to work better for more superficial wrinkles.

Filler Longevity and Reversibility: Some fillers last longer than others, depending on the type of filler, the area treated, and the individual patient's metabolism. In addition, an important consideration is that some fillers can be dissolved, but other types of fillers cannot. These factors can have an impact on filler choice.

Skin Elasticity and Overall Tone: Surgery might be a better option for patients who have extreme sagging skin or volume loss.

Facial Contours: The natural contours of a patient's face and their overall skin health will largely determine the chosen fillers injection depth and volume.

Dermal Fillers and Safety

The most important consideration when using dermal fillers is safety. There are three main points to consider:

1. The reputation of the medical practice you choose

2. The expertise of the clinician

3. The products that your clinician will use and whether they are right for you

There is a plethora of dermal fillers available on the market. They have a reputation for being extremely effective in replenishing the areas that have lost volume, to enhance your facial structure, to fill in the fine lines and wrinkles, and to help restore the fullness of the lips, cheeks, and maybe other areas on the face, such as tear troughs. Each type of dermal filler is used in different ways to enhance your facial volume and definition as well as to correct and restore facial contours.

The results that you can expect largely come down to the knowledge and experience of your clinician.

The table below lists the common areas where dermal fillers are used:

List of Common Areas Where Dermal FIllers are Used

Body Part	How Dermal Fillers are Used
Face	Worry lines across the forehead (dermal fillers are used in this area, and only if lines remain deep after complete relaxation with a neurotoxin) Smoker's lines around the mouth Nose to mouth folds Cheeks to restore firmness and volume Chin to improve tauness and firmness Jawline to improve tautness and firmness Under eye due to hollows or dark circles Smile lines Lines and volume loss around the eyes (crow's feet) Lip volume and border
Neck	Sagging jowels Neck lines Decolletage lines
Hands	Scars, skin laxity, popping veins

List of Common Fillers Used For Various Body Parts

Body Part	Dermal Fillers
Cheeks 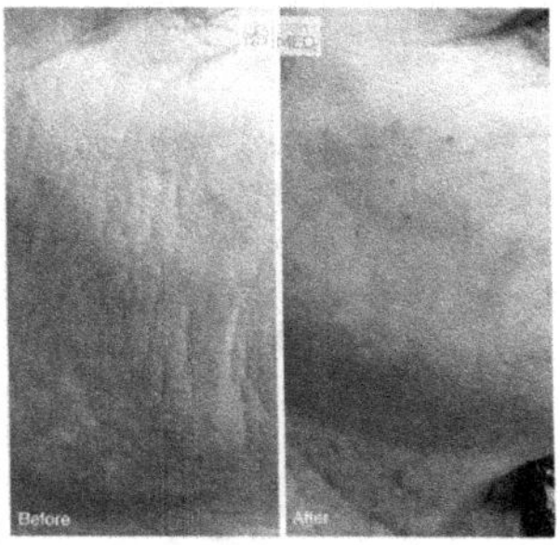	Juvderm Voluma Radiesse Sculptra
Ears	Juvederm Ultra/Ultra Plus Belotero Restylane Vollure
Corner of mouth 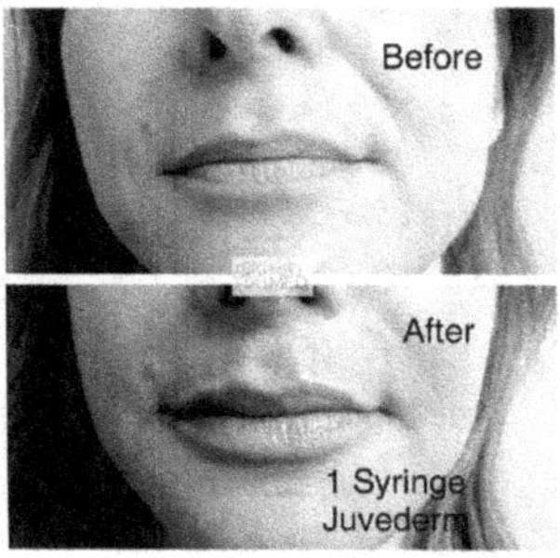	Vollure Voluma Restylane Juvederm Ultra/Ultra Plus

Body Part	Dermal Fillers	
Plumping of the lips and lip lines 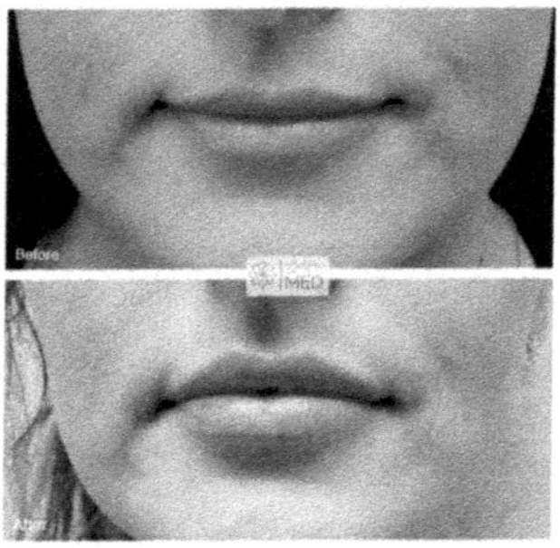	Juvederm Ultra Belotero Restylane Silk Volbella	
Chin, lower chin and pre-jowel	Juvederm Ultra/Ultra Plus Vollure Restylane Silk Restylane Radiesse	
Marionette	Juvederm Ultra/Ultra Plus Radiesse Restylane Vollure	
Naso-labial folds	Radiesse Restylane Juvederm Ultra Plus Vollure	Restylane Lyft Juvederm Ultra Juvederm Voluma Sculptra

Body Part	Dermal Fillers
Tear troughs 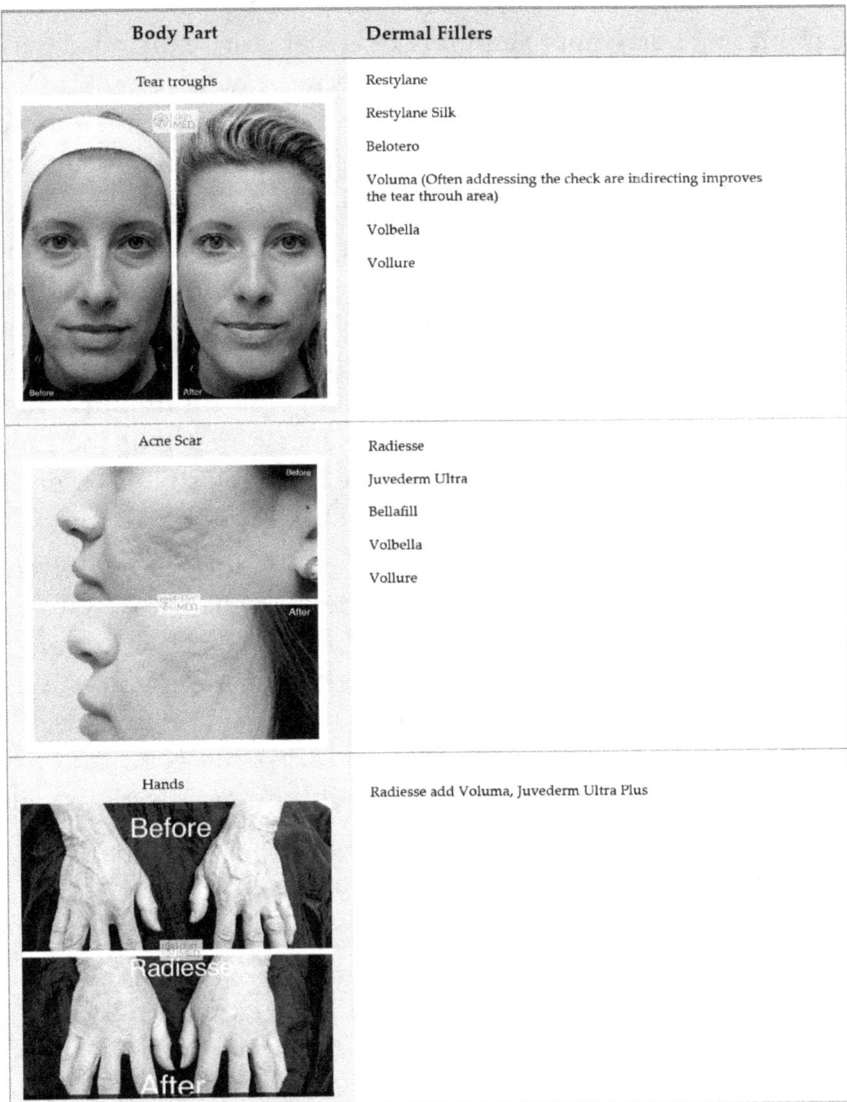	Restylane Restylane Silk Belotero Voluma (Often addressing the check are indirecting improves the tear throuh area) Volbella Vollure
Acne Scar	Radiesse Juvederm Ultra Bellafill Volbella Vollure
Hands	Radiesse add Voluma, Juvederm Ultra Plus

Please note: Frown lines and crow's feet would typically be treated with a product such as Botox.

Concluding Comments about Dermal Fillers

One point that I do want to emphasize is that you really need to do your research before you trust a skin specialist with your skin. Just because a dermal filler has been touted by someone on the Internet as the best possible treatment for aging skin, it does not mean that you should take what they say as gospel.

So, if you are considering dermal fillers, you are confused about your next step, and/or you are receiving conflicting information, you should consult with a reputable skin care specialist, such as a dermatologist or physician assistant/nurse practitioner who is trained and who specializes in dermatology, to figure out which type of dermal filler is right for you. Never forget that the most important issue with any skin procedure is safety, so it is essential that you choose someone whom you trust.

Nevertheless, given the potential for litigation if something went wrong, dermal fillers today are generally very safe. That does not mean though that you do not need to do your own research and ask questions. For example, pregnant women or women who are breast feeding are not advised to have this treatment, and if you have acne, it is a good idea to address the condition first because you may be prone to infection following injections with dermal fillers.

Also, there are also certain health conditions that render you unsuitable for treatments with these types of fillers, such as immune disease and rheumatoid arthritis.

Despite what you have read on the Internet or heard from a friend, there is not a dermal filler that best fits everyone. All dermal fillers have their pros and cons. Once again, the results you achieve largely come down to your clinician's experience, their knowledge, their skills, and their technique. Also, your body's tolerance to the substances used in dermal fillers needs to be taken into account. The best way to discover if fillers are for you is to speak to a qualified skin specialist who will discuss the types of dermal fillers available and identify which type of filler is best for you.

Summary of Key Points

- Dermal fillers are safe, painless, quick, and effective.
- Your clinician will customize each session to you.
- Dermal fillers achieve instantaneous results, giving you a softer, smoother face.
- The results will help restore and enhance your looks giving you a fresher and more natural appearance.
- Your facial expressions will be unaffected.
- There is very little down-time or recovery time—so you can get a session and no one will know.
- They are a natural alternative to an invasive surgery.
- Depending on the product used, the effects are usually long-lasting, but not permanent.

Take Charge of Your Beauty

CHAPTER SIX

Skin Therapy

This chapter provides some guidelines about the things you need to consider before purchasing skincare products. There is information overload on the Internet, some of which is contradictory, confusing, and misleading. One of the first things I tell my clients when they ask me about the best skincare products on the market is that there is no single product that works well for everyone.

Nevertheless, there are some general guidelines that can help you to choose a product that works for your skin, and hopefully this chapter will provide you with some helpful advice to help you narrow down your search for products that work well for your skin.

Skin Cleansers

It is particularly important to adopt a good skincare routine as early as possible, and a good skincare routine begins with choosing the right cleanser for your skin type.

Cleansers have an important function in keeping your skin fresh, and choosing the right cleanser ensures that your other skincare products perform maximally. For instance, using a good cleanser will allow other beauty treatments, including moisturizers, to work more effectively. Nevertheless, although cleansing is very important, it is essential that you do not over clean your skin.

You should generally wash your face no more than twice a day: once in the morning to remove oil and bacteria and once in the evening to remove makeup, sunscreen, and grime. It is imperative that you use water that is either lukewarm or room temperature rather than very hot or cold water because using extreme temperatures on your skin can cause redness and broken capillaries.

Picking the right cleanser for your skin type can feel a bit overwhelming, so the next section will make things a bit easier by explaining what to look for in a cleanser according to your skin type.

To Pick the Right Cleanser for Your Skin, Consider the Following Questions:

Is the cleanser too drying?

Does the cleanser remove makeup and take off sunscreen?

Does it have any ingredients that I should avoid, such as sodium lauryl sulfate or alcohol?

Your cleanser needs to be strong enough to clean, but not so harsh that it leaves your skin feeling dry. It does need to remove dirt and grime, but it is important that it does not strip away all of your skin's oil, which acts as a natural defense. As a rule, if you use a cleanser that makes your skin feel either tight or squeaky, it is too harsh. Similarly, you won't know whether a cleanser will clean well unless you try it yourself.

A good cleanser is one that removes the things that have to be removed, such as dirt, sunscreen, and makeup, but leaves behind the skin's natural oils.

Steps for Choosing the Right Cleanser

1. Check to see whether the cleanser is suitable for your skin type. For instance, if a cleanser is recommended for dry skin and you have dry skin, that cleanser will probably be too drying for you.

2. Check the product ingredients to see whether the cleanser contains harsh detergents. If there are harsh ingredients, such as sodium laureth sulfate (SLES) or alcohol, and these ingredients appear high up on the ingredient list, it is best to avoid that product.

3. Read product reviews to see what other people think of the product you are thinking of buying. It is important to look for reviews that warn about adverse skin reactions, for instance. If you can, obtain a sample of the product and try it before you commit to spending your money on it.

4. Test the product on your skin. If the product leaves your skin feeling taut and dry, or oily, it is best to look elsewhere for a product that is more suitable for your skin type. You can test it on a small portion of your forearm if you have a history of being sensitive before placing it all over your face. Alternatively, you can also test the product by using small amounts of the product on specific areas of the face.

If your skin is on the drier side, avoid foaming cleansers, and instead, choose products that are designed to be moisturizing; but if your skin is on the oily side, foaming cleansers are often a good choice. If you have sensitive skin, try avoiding cleansers with acids, fragrances, dyes, and other harsh ingredients.

If you have acne, it does not necessarily mean that you should use a harsh cleanser. Removing excessive oil can sometimes help, but that is not always the case. If a cleanser dries out your skin, it is important to stop using it because it is likely to make the problem worse.

A General Description of the Different Skin Cleansers for Various Skin Types

Bar Soap

Bar soaps are generally not recommended for any skin type because they are made from strong ingredients that are designed to remove everything from your skin, including the skin's natural oils.

Foaming Cleansers

Foaming cleansers tend to be drying, so they are generally best for oily skin types, but even the gentlest foaming cleansers should be avoided for skin types that are prone to drying. Foaming cleansers can also be found in the form of gels and creams. Cream foaming cleansers contain oils and emollients that are less drying than foaming cleansers.

Non-Foaming

Non-foaming cleansers are often marketed as gentle skin cleansers and are generally advertised as being for people who have sensitive skin. These are mild cleansers that do not foam, but they are often ineffective at removing sunscreen and makeup. They are a good option to use in the morning for people with dry skin.

Cleansing Balms

Cleansing balms are either cream or oil-based products that are removed with either tissues or makeup pads. They are often used as makeup removers, particularly by people who have dry skin. Cream cleansing balms are like cold creams, and oil balms resemble petroleum jelly that are solid at room temperature, but they liquefy when they come into contact with the skin. Cleansing balms are particularly effective for removing heavy makeup, sunscreen, and waterproof products. They usually leave an oily residue after they are removed with tissues or makeup pads, but they can be used in conjunction with other cleansers.

Water Cleansers

Water cleansers are also referred to as micellar cleansers, and as the name suggests, they are water-based. They are similar to cleansing toners. The cleansing solution is generally applied to a cotton pad, then applied to the skin, and is removed with either a clean cotton pad or rinsed off with water. Water cleansers are generally very gentle, so they are suitable for people with sensitive skin.

Oil Cleansers

Cleansing oils are designed to remove makeup and water-proof sunscreen. These products are used by applying one or two pumps of cleansing oil to dry skin, which is then either rubbed off with a cotton pad or washed off with water. Oil cleansers tend to be moisturizing, so they are a good option for people with dry or mature skin.

Medicated Cleansers

Medicated cleansers are usually foam cleansers that are tailored for acne-prone skin, particularly teenagers. The active ingredients of these cleaners are often salicylic acid, which helps to unclog pores, and benzoyl peroxide, which helps to eradicate bacteria. These types of cleansers are too drying for most skin types, and gentle cleansers are often a better option for people who have acne-prone skin because stripping the skin too much can exacerbate some acne.

Soap-Free Cleansers

Soap-free cleansers do not contain either sodium lauryl sulfate or sodium laureth sulfate. Soap-free cleansers are a good option for people with dry or sensitive skin, and they are the cleanser of choice to use about a week before getting a chemical peel because they prepare the skin and make the peel more effective.

Overall, the best cleanser for you will depend on your skin type. It needs to adequately clean your skin, without stripping it or drying it out too much. In general, it is better to choose a cleanser that is too gentle than one that is too harsh.

Over-the-Counter vs. Prescription Cleansers

Most cleansers, creams, and body products on the market fall into the category of over-the-counter, and these are products that you can easily find in drugstores, department stores, and supermarkets. These products range in price from budget-friendly to very expensive although they all contain similar concentrations of pure ingredients due to American Food and Drug Association regulations, which is approximately 70 percent.

Over-the-counter products tend to contain very few active ingredients because they are generally marketed for most skin types. Therefore, the vast majority of their ingredients are inactive compounds, preservatives, stabilizers, and fragrances.

Pharmaceutical skincare products are classified as drugs. Pharmaceutical skincare products constitute less than five percent of all skincare products although they are the most effective of all skincare products. These products can only be obtained from licensed professions, and because they are regulated by the FDA, they must meet stringent criteria: They have to be made of 99.9 percent pure active ingredients; they need to be backed up by scientific studies; and they need to have proven positive, enhancing effects on the skin. For instance, they have to have proven efficacy in reducing the appearance of wrinkles, diminishing the appearance of age spots, firming and plumping the skin, and providing effective hydration.

Which products are the best? The difference between over-the-counter products and pharmaceuticals is the quality and proportion of active ingredients, and pharmaceuticals have far more of both. Also, over-the-counter products are chosen by the individual consumer themselves whereas pharmaceuticals are chosen by a licensed professionals for optimal results.

Skin Moisturizers

Choosing a moisturizer that is right for your skin can seem overwhelming. During the summer months, your skin tends to need a lighter moisturizer, but a hydrating moisturizer is often needed for the drying months of winter.

You probably have your own preferences and ideas about moisturizers, but you should know how a good moisturizer should feel when you apply it, what it contains, whether it should take time to soak into the skin, as well as whether it is right for your skin type.

Generally, moisturizers contain four main ingredients: 1) occlusives, which are like white petrolatum and form a protective shield over the skin; 2) humectants, such as hyaluronic acid, which are designed to draw in water from the deeper skin layers; 3) emollients, such as glycerine, which fill in cracks and reduce roughness between skin cells; and 4) barrier-repair products, such as ceramides, which replace natural fats and promote optimal skin function.

Regardless of Your Skin Type, Your Moisturizer Should Do the Following:

- It should glide effortlessly on your skin and make your skin feel soft. A common moisturizer ingredient that achieves this is dimethicone, which provides a protective barrier on the surface of the skin so that water cannot escape and environmental pollutants are blocked from getting in. Dimethicone is often used in conjunction with mineral or other oils, such as jojoba oil.

- It should contain an NMF (natural moisturizing factor) . These are molecules that allow the moisturizer to reach the outer layer of the skin in order to provide deeper moisturizing.

- A high-quality product will absorb quickly, and it will not leave your skin feeling greasy. It should feel light and hydrate the skin so that it feels soft.

- Quality moisturizers should also be unscented although the consistency that you choose should depend on your skin type. For example, a gel would be a better choice for oily skin, lotion is often adequate for combination skin, while a rich cream is often more suitable for dry and-or mature skin.

In general, a quality moisturizer will immediately plump the skin and smooth fine lines. When you consistently use a good moisturizer, your skin barrier will repair itself, and it should be less sensitive. Also, a quality product will often normalize the production of oil, so that your skin is more even.

So, What Type of Moisturizer Is Right for You?

No single moisturizer works for everyone. This means that you will need to evaluate various products to find a moisturizer that best suits you. It can also be useful to speak to a skin specialist for advice about products that would work best for you.

Best Moisturizers for Dry Skin

If you suffer from dry skin, then it is useful to look for certain ingredients that specifically treat dry skin. For example, humectants lock in water. Also, look for products that contain emollients, which are used to soothe and soften the skin.

It is important to note that a thicker formula is not necessarily always the best option for dry skin. Sometimes creams are manufactured to be thicker to give wearers a feeling of luxury. Petrolatum products, occlusives, and mineral oils should be mostly avoided as moisturizers because most of them tend to sit on top of the skin and clog pores.

In addition, surfactants, such as sodium lauryl sulfate, are very drying on dry skin, so they should also be avoided.

Best Moisturizer for Oily Skin

If your skin is particularly oily, you might need to use a product that has mattifying properties to reduce the appearance of oiliness. Light-weight, oil-free, and water-based moisturizers are recommended for skin that is prone to oiliness, and rich creams and hydrating formulas that contain oils should be avoided.

The Active Ingredients in Skincare Products

The following ingredients are some of the most commonly used active ingredients in skincare products:

Alpha Hydroxy Acids (AHA)

Alpha hydroxy acids (AHAs) are a class of chemical compounds that are naturally contained in sugar cane, milk, and fruit. Although they are called acids, they should not be confused with industrial acids, such as sulfuric acid. The AHAs most commonly used in cosmetic products are glycolic acid (a derivative of sugar cane) and lactic acid. Other examples of AHAs used in skincare products are citric acid, hydroxyoctanoic acid, and hydroxydecanoic acid. These acids can be either extracted from natural sources or synthetically manufactured.

Glycolic Acid

Glycolic acid is an alpha hydroxy acid. It is a product that is extracted from sugar cane. Glycolic acid is the most commonly used alpha hydroxy acid, and it is considered to be among the safest. Gycolic acid has many benefits: It removes dead skin cells, and it also smooths fine lines. With continued use, the size of the skin's pores is often reduced, and it can also help to reduce and eliminate acne. With long-term use, the general condition of the skin tends to improve and pigmentation often fades or disappears completely. Glycolic acid penetrates into the dermis of the skin, which is the skin's deepest layer. The dermis is where collagen and elastin are manufactured. Glycolic acid products will plump the skin as well as reduce the appearance of fine lines and wrinkles.

Beta-Hydroxy Acid (Salicylic Acid)

Salicylic acid removes dead skin, and it is also used to improve the texture and color of sun-damaged skin. Salicylic acid penetrates oil-laden hair follicle openings, so it is also sometimes used for people with acne. There are numerous skincare products on the market that contain this ingredient, and some of them are available over-the-counter although prescription versions contain higher concentrations of it. Research on salicylic acid has found that it is less irritating than alpha hydroxy acids although it does provide similar improvements in the skin's texture and color.

Growth Factors

Growth factors are proteins that regulate cellular growth and promote cell proliferation and cell differentiation. They have an important role in the maintenance of healthy skin.

Growth factors are naturally secreted skin cells of the epidermis (the skin's outer layer) and the dermis (the skin later that sits between the epidermis and subcutaneous skin tissue).

Growth factors stimulate skin tissue in its repair and regeneration, and they promote the production of collagen and elastic fibres, which give skin its smoothness. Growth factors also stimulate the biochemical pathways that promote skin tissue repair and regeneration. The interaction of numerous growth factors with other proteins is what promotes skin repair.

Skin creams that contain growth factors are sometimes used in skincare creams. These skin creams usually contain a mixture of growth factors and other proteins, which are designed to slow down intrinsic skin aging (i.e., natural aging) and extrinsic skin aging, which is caused by environmental factors.

Growth factors have empirical value in reducing the appearance of fine lines and wrinkles, fading, and the appearance of age spots and blotchy skin. They also have the ability to enhance skin elasticity and texture, and promote smoothness and firmer skin.

Some products that contain growth factors are available over-the-counter although the quality and strength of these growth factors are significantly less than those contained in prescription-only products. The over-the-counter products do not have FDA approval.

Stem Cells

Stem cells are one category of active ingredients used in advanced prescription skincare products. Stem cells are an advanced skincare solution, and they are proven to be safe although there has been some confusion and controversy about their use.

Plant stem cells, instead of human stem cells, are a preferable option because they provide numerous benefits in the treatment of many skin conditions, but they do not create the same controversies inherent in the extraction and use of human stem cells. Malus Domestica (Swiss apple), Vitis Vinifera (grapefruit), and Syringa Vulgaris (lilac leaf) are among the most popular stem cells used in skincare products.

Stem cells have many benefits, and they are especially useful in the treatment of inflammation, aging, and sun damage. Stem cell technology has now advanced to an extent that it may soon be possible to replace rather than repair damaged skin cells. Further research into advanced product formulations that look at the mechanisms of stem cells in skin rejuvenation will allow skincare professionals to provide tailored skincare treatments that offer the best options and results for every patient.

Skin Bleaching Creams

Skin bleaching creams are usually used by dermatologists and other skincare professionals to lighten specific areas of the skin, such as pigmentation, age spots, acne scars, or discoloration due to hormonal factors. Skin bleaching creams are marketed under numerous names, including skin whiteners and brighteners, and fading creams. The way they work is that they stop the skin's production of melanin, which in turn, lightens the skin.

There are several different ingredients that can be used to lighten the skin, but the most commonly used in the United States is hydroquinone. This drug is strictly regulated by the FDA, and therefore, concentrations above two percent are prescription-only.

Other skin bleaching creams contain either steroids or retinoic acid while others use natural ingredients, such as kojic acid or arbutin. Arbutin is a naturally-produced derivative of hydroquinone that is found in plants, such as blueberries and cranberries, and it is often present in combination with other skin-lightening ingredients, while kojic acid is an antioxidant derived from a fungus. It breaks down the melanin to prevent further production of melatonin. Both of these products are available in over-the-counter skincare products although they tend to be poorer quality and in weaker concentrations than prescription-only products.

Precaution with these products is critical because of the potential risks of using these products. Consequently, people who are affected by hyperpigmentation should consult a qualified skin professional for professional advice and treatment.

Retinals and Retinoids

Retinals and retinoids are designed to reverse the signs of aging. Each has proven effectiveness in the reduction of wrinkles, in improving acne, boosting collagen, and improving overall skin tone.

Retinoids are chemical compounds that resemble vitamin A, and they work by removing old skin cells and boosting new cellular growth. In addition, they promote collagen production and reduce pigmentation. The type and strength of retinoid that you should use on your skin largely depends on the type of skin condition you are treating, your skin type, and your age.

Retinol is also a form of vitamin A, but it naturally occurs in the skin. When it is applied to the skin topically, the enzymes of the skin convert it to retinoic acid. These products have proven efficacy in reducing the appearance of fine lines and discoloration, which are clinically proven to reduce the appearance of lines, improve discoloration issues, and revitalize the skin.

Retinols are better for some skin types while retinoids are better for others. For some people, just applying retinol on a daily basis over an extended period of time produces optimal results while in other people, better results will be obtained with a prescription-only retinoid.

What Is Organic Skincare and What Do I Need to Know About It?

The words "organic" and "natural" now have a cult following in the diet world, so when these words started appearing in skincare, it created significant confusion for people. While the idea of natural and organic products does have some intuitive appeal, products that are labelled as such and which meet the criteria for being organic products are rarely going to give you the same results as non-organic products.

Something I stress to my clients often is that natural and organic products can often cause significant irritation and allergies because they tend to contain large quantities of essential oils and botanical ingredients. The problem is that public perception is too often skewed by the media.

However, the media rarely points out that organic and natural ingredients are not always safe or effective to use on your skin. For example, there are some natural compounds that are used in some organic and natural products, which in large quantities, can be carcinogenic. Therefore, buying organic food and buying organic skincare products are two very different things. In fact, one of the difficulties with organic skincare products is that they are not regulated in the same way as organic foods.

The claim that natural cosmetics are better for the skin has not been proven in clinical studies. While some people might use products that are labelled as "organic" or "natural" due to an allergy to chemical ingredients or preservatives, you are just as likely to be allergic to a product that is natural. Therefore, product labels that use the words "organic" or "natural" can be quite misleading.

The FDA does not regulate skincare products until the product is on the market, and while the FDA does inspect products for safety, these skin products are not as regulated as diligently as drugs and food.

It is also important to be aware that a skincare manufacturer can add two natural ingredients and then market the product as "containing natural ingredients," but be aware that it might also contain synthetic dyes, chemicals, and fillers. Also, even if a number of ingredients in the product are derived from natural sources, synthetic chemicals are still often used in the manufacturing of the product.

Additionally, "natural" does not always necessarily mean safe. Bacterial contamination is natural, and it is not a chemical, but you would not put it on your face. Poison ivy is also natural, but again, it should not go on your face. Bananas have great nutritional value, but applying it to your face will not protect you from the sun's ultraviolet rays, nor will it moisturize or protect your skin from environmental irritants.

So, the overall message in regards to organic skincare is that it is far preferable to do your own research; rather than looking for the words "natural" and "organic," look at the specific ingredients in the product instead.

Take Charge of Your Beauty

CHAPTER SEVEN

My Skin Has Changed —Help Me!

Let's talk about acne, which is a very unpopular skin condition. Why? According, to the *Journal of American Academy of Dermatology*, 54 percent of women older than 25 have some facial acne.

Acne during adulthood is far harder to treat than the pimples that most of us had in our adolescence. Globally, outbreaks of adult acne have been on the rise in recent years. Some of the women I have treated for adult acne have said that they never had as much as a pimple in the past, yet they have found themselves dealing with adult acne.

If you have ever suffered acne at any stage during your life, I am sure you will agree that it can be distressing. One possible reason why acne is on the rise in women specifically is due to unprecedentedly high levels of stress. As already mentioned, we are living and working longer than anyone ever did in yesteryears. The normal daily stressors to maintain an income, combined with workplace stress, poor diet, and environmental stressors, can impact the condition of the skin. Also, skincare products that contain irritants, some pharmaceuticals, and inevitable hormonal changes throughout the lifespan can take a significant toll on the skin.

Acne and acne scarring are among the most anxiety-provoking skin conditions for clients that I have treated over the years. Because the condition of our skin has so much to do with the overall state of our physical and mental health, many people have turned to psycho-dermatology for answers.

What is psycho-dermatology? Psycho-dermatology treats skin conditions by addressing the connection between mind and body and via treating skin conditions that are aggravated by psychological or emotional stress. It is a comparatively new discipline of psychosomatic medicine. The theory of this treatment is that emotions, for example, stress and anxiety, trigger some skin conditions. It is universally accepted that the skin, as our largest organ, is affected by our brain and nervous system.

For instance, if we feel scared, we might break into a cold sweat, or if we are embarrassed, we might blush. In much the same way, stress can trigger a rush of the hormone testosterone, which leads to the production of excess oil in the sebaceous glands. This excess oil is one of the contributing factors of acne. Additionally, chronic stress causes the adrenal glands to over-produce cortisol, which then slows the process of healing. Psycho-dermatology clinicians will typically combine antibiotics or topical medications with talking methods, such as cognitive behavioral therapy (CBT).

If you choose to see your general practitioner about your acne, they will invariably offer a range of prescription drugs that target the main causes of acne. However, while skin specialists, such as dermatologists, will likely suggest the same course of medications, they have more experience monitoring skin conditions. Also, skin specialists can offer a broader range of options to treat your acne other than medication.

As you may be aware, there are a range of topical treatments, prescription and non-prescription medications available for the treatment of acne. I have highlighted some of the main ones that are used:

Oral antibiotics can be classed as moderately effective when it comes to treating acne, and in the past antibiotics were often the general practitioner's treatment of choice. The antibiotics were usually prescribed over the course of several months, or even years in more chronic cases.

In recent years, doctors have been reluctant to prescription oral antibiotics due to bacterial resistance, and also, some of the newer antibiotics tend to be less well tolerated by the body, some antibiotics can be expensive, and there are antibiotics that are not readily accessible in many countries. Therefore, a good topical antibiotic, which also has antibacterial and anti-inflammatory effects, is suggested because they tend to be better tolerated. A common course of treatment would be to use a topical antibiotic in conjunction with benzoyl peroxide.

Benzoyl Peroxide is generally accepted as a very effective acne treatment, and it is a product that needs to be used regularly in order to be effective. Benzoyl peroxide increases the rate at which skin cells are removed (which helps to unblock pores), it also very effectively reduces inflammation, and it suppresses the bacteria that encourages acne to spread. So, it works by killing bacteria while exfoliating your pores. That said, benzyl peroxide is not the gentlest of products, so I strongly recommend that you use it only on the affected areas; otherwise it can irritate your skin and cause it to become very dry.

Salicylic Acid is used in a large amount of treatments and cleansers. It is also referred to as beta-hydroxy acid. When it is applied topically, it can slows down the shedding of the cells inside your follicles, which then effectively works to exfoliate your skin and prevent clogging. It softens keratin, a protein which forms part of the structure of the skin. It is far less irritating than benzoyl peroxide, and it is gentle enough for your entire face. If you are plagued by blackheads and spots, but no deep, closed comedones (whiteheads), then salicylic acid could be a good choice, but be aware not to over use it.

AHA glycolic acid helps acne, and it also helps wrinkles. Be mindful that the product you choose must be at the right pH level to be effective, and also not all skin types respond well to AHA treatments. Glycolic acid is the smallest of the AHAs, and one of its benefits is that it penetrates the skin faster and far more effectively when it is used on mild acne rather than on severe acne. From a topical application of AHA glycolic acid, the most commonly reported side effects are skin irritation, peeling, redness, and scaling although the side effects tend to disappear about two weeks after the treatment. Caution needs to be diligently maintained with this treatment because excessively or incorrectly applying AHA can burn the skin and cause permanent damage.

Retinols are used extensively, and they tend to be very effective. Retinols are a vitamin A derivative, and when the skin absorbs it, it's converted to retinoic acid. If you have skin that has severe sun damage or you suffer from comedonal acne, you will very likely get better results from using a prescription retinoid treatment. If you have not used retinols before or have just started to use them, remember to start slowly by incorporating the product into your nighttime regime, and use it sparingly every second night. Why at night? Basically, sunlight deactivates retinoic acid, which then renders it useless. If you have sensitive skin or are unsure, then mix it in with your usual moisturizer to minimize any irritation. As part of your regime, try using the retinol on the tops of your hands, your neck, and your chest. Be aware that if you wax any skin surface that you intend to use retinols on, then you need to abstain from using the retinol for a couple of days before and after your wax! Be mindful not to get carried away with retinols. A pea-sized amount is ample.

Spironolactone is an incredibly effective medicine, particularly for adult women with hormonal acne. It is generally a safe choice when prescribed under the care of a knowledgeable professional who will also be likely to suggest a well-balanced diet and sufficient hydration when on this medication. You need to be very aware that spironolactone can produce birth defects, and it should, therefore, not be used during pregnancy or if you are intending to become pregnant. For most people, it will take up to 3 months before you hit the titration levels, at which stage you will notice optimal benefits. A possible side effect of this medication is irregular periods. To reduce potential side effects, your skin specialist should start you on a smaller dose and carefully increase your dosage under regular supervision. If you suffer from moderate or severe acne, then higher doses would be required to achieve the desired effect. If you notice the side effects outweigh the benefits, speak with your skin specialist to discuss alternatives.

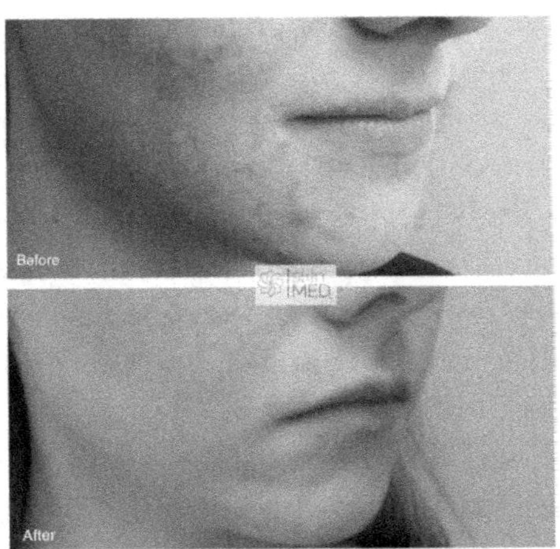

Skin Changes across the Lifespan

Who doesn't want to have a better understanding of the effects of aging and what can help? Let's have a quick look at what happens to our skin as we age. If we face the reality of it as soon as possible, then how we look in our thirties and beyond very much depends on how we have looked after our skin up until then and how we look after it in future. Let's face it: Everyone wants to have youthful-looking skin. Despite the best marketing efforts and the wildest claims about expensive skincare products, intrinsic and extrinsic aging are an inevitable part of getting older. That said, there are definite steps that we can all take to ensure we look healthy, and as wrinkle- and blemish-free as possible for longer.

We have already talked about treatments, such as Botox and dermal fillers, so let's have a brief look at the key changes that happen during each decade from our thirties.

Thirties: Environmental damage from pollution, sunlight, and smoke starts taking a noticeable toll on your skin by the age of 30, which commonly results in the loosening of collagen fibers, looser skin, fine lines, and wrinkles. When you smile, subcutaneous fat forms ridges that refuse to bounce back as readily as they did at the age of twenty. You may also notice more fine lines around key areas, such as your eyes. If you smoke, the pursing of your lips will exaggerate any lines that you have around the mouth. You might also start to lose some of your skin tone because the elastic support from your lymph glands (responsible for flushing out toxins) starts to weaken. This can lead to puffiness around the eyes, and the overall complexion of your skin can become less bright. With all of that, you might notice weight changes, and possibly more cellulite, for example. This is due to hormonal changes, which is perfectly normal: The blood and lymph circulation will start to slow, and fat tends to accumulate around the bottom, thighs, and hips. You might also notice the development of stretch marks.

What can you do? Stepping up your exercise regime is very beneficial for your entire body and mind, and muscle atrophy is likely to be slowed with regular exercise and via maintaining a healthy balanced diet of fresh fruits, vegetables, grains, and fish, which are all high in antioxidants. It is very important to maintain hydration to retain moisture in the skin tissue, sun protection for your skin is absolutely critical, and you should also ensure that you get enough quality sleep. Ramp up your anti-aging skin regimen, especially at night when skin rests and repairs, and consider adding a product containing retinol, which thickens skin by increasing collagen production to smooth wrinkles and reverse volume loss. Exfoliation is as important as ever to rid the complexion of skin-dulling dead cells and a good eye cream or serum can help to keep fine lines and dark circles at bay. Treat yourself to a nourishing face mask whenever your skin feels in need of an extra boost, and invest in a good skin brightener for instant radiance.

Forties: It is very common for your lymphatic system to slow down during your forties. This is how your body gets rid of toxins, but slower lymphatic drainage can cause puffiness around your eyes and cheeks. Our forties are a time when hormones, such as estrogen, start to decline, which can cause your skin to sag and wrinkle around the neck and chest. It is perfectly normal to see signs of tiredness at this age, and of course, life's stressors and excesses are reflected in our faces all too often. If you do not look after yourself, the signs of excessive alcohol can lead to dilated blood vessels, creating a red/blushed appearance. If you are smoking, it may break down your collagen and dehydrate the watery gel inside your skin that is responsible for keeping your skin plump and elastic. Naturally, environmental factors, such as too much sun, may give your skin a mottled, uneven, or leathery appearance. There can also be signs of substantial drying and dulling of your skin. The loss of volume in the face leads to hollowing or sunken-looking eyes and slackening skin due to estrogen-related bone loss that is starting to affect your facial structure, resulting in more visible wrinkles, capillaries, broken blood vessels, and age spots. My clients who are in the forties often tell me, "My skin changed overnight"! This is true. Dramatic changes take place in our forties, particularly when it comes to loss of volume and elasticity in our face.

Action: The good news is that there are quite a few things that you can do to visibly improve the way your skin looks and feels. Although we cannot stop the aging process entirely, there is still plenty you can do. For example, massaging your skin when applying moisturizers helps to drain your lymphatic fluid. Healthy lifestyle choices, like staying hydrated, getting adequate sleep, eating a balanced diet of whole, unprocessed foods, and exercising, will help improve your look, too. Sebum production will slow down in our forties, so it is important to choose quality skincare that is rich, nourishing, and moisturizing. Also, there are a range of skin-firming treatments that you can receive from a skincare specialist. At this age, you might also consider upgrading to a prescription retinol, such as retinoic acid or Retin-A, and if you have done so already, maybe increase the concentration of the product you use. Retinol helps your skin to behave as it did when you were younger and healthier—it reduces wrinkles, thickens skin, and can help control acne. Your doctor or dermatologist may also suggest a course of phytoestrogens into your regime. Phytoestrogens help by mimicking estrogen's collagen, which aids in restoring our skin.

Fifties: The signs of both intrinsic and extrinsic aging will become more prevalent once you turn fifty. If you have not taken regular exercise, you will also see the effects in loss of tone and muscle. Like the majority of us, if you if you have ever been on a diet in your life, your skin will lose much of its ability to regain its elasticity between periods of rapid weight gain and loss, thus becoming thinner, drier, deflating, and loosening. Our facial lines become deeper, our pores stretch, eye lids may sag and become hooded, or our eye sockets hollow. A very common complaint is that spider veins may become more visible. Of course, age spots show up, and if you didn't already have it, you might begin to get facial hair on the cheeks, chin, and upper lip. Once you reach menopause, your estrogen production will significantly slow down (usually at around 51–52 years old). You will lose up to one third of your collagen within the first three to five years of menopause, depending on your physiology. This will result in a loss of the skin's moisture and radiance. You can also expect that inflammation will increase dramatically in some cases, making skin more vulnerable to environmental damage. Your skin is also more likely to become more dehydrated than in earlier years, resulting in further weakening of your skin's collagen and elastin.

Action: In our fifties, many of us feel that the clock is ticking, and it is at this stage that many people seek the help of skincare specialists for injectables, lasers, radio-frequency, or ultrasound treatments. Botox smooths lines and dermal fillers, such as the ones discussed in previous chapters (i.e., Juvéderm, Juvéderm Voluma, Belotero, and Radiesse), can be used to fill in deeper grooves and replace lost plumpness. Restylane injections can be used to camouflage dark circles while laser treatments can fade or erase brown spots. Radio-frequency treatments and ultrasound wave procedures can tighten skin in areas like the brow, neck, and chest. There might be a time in your fifties that your doctor recommends hormone therapy to help raise your estrogen levels, which is a safe option for many women.

In regard to skincare products, the fifties is definitely the time to concentrate on ensuring the skin is adequately moisturized because without the natural hyaluronic acid that comes with estrogen, skin doesn't hold onto moisture. Moisture is more important than ever, and nourishing masks and/or serums will help a lot in keeping your complexion looking healthy and hydrated. A night cream can also work wonders on dry skin while you sleep. Many of my clients in this age range tell me their skin is so dry that it is literally cracking. If this is happening, then you need to stop using harsh cleaners, such as soaps or foaming cleaners, try reducing the amount of showers that you take, try to only wash your face during your nighttime routine to avoid breaching low levels of hydration in your skin, choose products that have hyaluronic acid in them, which will help to reduce any irritation, and look at using skin barrier-supporting ceramides.

In closing, the take-home message is that there is plenty you can do during the lifecycle to maximize and enhance a youthful and radiant you, and it's never too late to start.

CHAPTER EIGHT

Erase the Years Using Laser and Other Fun Devices!

The word "laser" is an acronym that stands for llight amplification by the stimulated emission of radiation. The first lasers that were used to treat skin conditions were introduced approximately 40 years ago, and among the first of these lasers were argon and carbon dioxide lasers, which were used to treat hemangiomas (a collection of small blood vessels that form a lump underneath the skin) and benign vascular birthmarks.

Nevertheless, although these types of lasers can effectively lighten birthmarks, there was a high risk of scarring. Over the past few decades, there has been significant progress made in laser therapy technology, and this has meant that laser is now an effective treatment for a whole host of skin conditions, including tattoo removal, as well as the treatment of scars, wrinkles, and pigmentation. In fact, in contemporary dermatology, there are numerous laser and light treatments that can be used for both rejuvenation and resurfacing.

Laser light works by focusing on small spots with a very high energy source. The process works via excitation of the molecules of the laser medium, which leads to the release of a photon of light. The objective of laser treatment is to destroy the target cells without adversely affecting surrounding tissue. Short pulses of laser reduce the amount that the damaged cells heat up, thereby reducing thermal injury that could result in scarring. Automated scanners are used to reduce the chance of targeting treatments areas more than once.

What Types of Lasers Are There?

There are several types of lasers that are used by modern skin specialists, and among the most common are the quasi-CW mode lasers and pulsed lasers.

The wavelength peaks of the laser light, pulse durations, and how the target skin tissue absorbs this determine the clinical applications of the laser types.

What Skin Conditions Can Be Treated with Lasers?

Vascular Lesions

Lasers are used to treat a broad category of vascular lesions, including birthmarks, broken capillaries, non-cancerous conditions of the cutaneous blood vessels, and other types of benign skin growths. Yellow-light quasi-CW laser and pulsed laser therapies are the most common because they minimize scarring and damage to surrounding tissue.

The pulsed dye laser is the preferred laser for most vascular lesions because of its clinical efficacy and low-risk. It can target areas of between 5 and 10mm, which allows fast treatment of large lesions. Side effects include bruising that can last up to two weeks as well as temporary changes in pigmentation.

Vascular lesions that have superficial blood vessels respond better to treatment than deeper and larger blood vessels, and consequently, it is advisable to start treatment as early as possible. In general, 80 percent fading of these vascular lesions can be achieved with an average of ten treatments, and follow-up treatments might be required if the lesion reappears.

Pigmented Lesions and Tattoos

QS lasers are effective at lightening or removing pigmentation, including age spots, birthmarks, and tattoos. The effectiveness of this type of laser treatment depends on the color of the lesion and its depth: superficial pigmentation tends to respond better to lasers that have a shorter wavelength while removal of deeper pigmentation is more effectively achieved by using lasers that have a longer wavelength. If you have darker skin, there is a risk from this treatment of hypopigmentation (lighter patches of skin) and hyperpigmentation (darker patches of skin), so your skin specialist needs to exercise caution when using this type of laser on your skin.

Tattoo pigmentation can be effectively removed with QS lasers, and this can be achieved without inflicting a lot of damage to the surrounding skin. Nevertheless, there is risk of scarring with this type of treatment.

Facial Wrinkles, Scars, and Sun-Damaged Skin

Facial laser resurfacing uses high-energy, pulsed, and scanned lasers.

Pulsed CO_2 lasers are considered to be the golden standard of facial rejuvenation, and they are effective in the treatment of sun damage, scars and wrinkles. On average, a fifty percent improvement is achieved by using this type of laser treatment. There are some side-effects of receiving CO_2 laser treatments, and these side effects include short-term tenderness, redness and swelling, and some scarring is also possible. Significant precaution needs to be exercised when treating darker skin with this type of laser, because it can result in either hyper or hypopigmentation. Erbium:YAG is another type of laser treatment that has been found to produce similar results to pulsed CO2 laser treatment, and it has been found to yield equally impressive results with similar side effects.

Crepey Skin

In the treatment of crepey skin, CO2 laser treatments send a beam of light deep into the layers of the skin. The laser works by irritating the deeper layers of the skin. After this process, the skin starts to heal, which results in an increase in collagen production. C02 lasers are not necessarily always a good option because they do require more downtime.

In more recent years, fractional lasers have become a popular option because they are less invasive. Fractional lasers are considered to be a better treatment for people who are under the age of 50, people who have mild to moderate acne scarring, and people who have fine lines. However, even though C02 are more invasive and require more down-time, they do tend to be a better option for older people, people who have deeper acne scarring, and people who require skin tightening.

Treatments for Sagging Skin

Radio frequency machines help boost collagen are considered to be good options for the treatment of sagging skin. These types of treatments stimulate the production of collagen in the body, which tightens the skin and restores some of the skin's lost elasticity. They can be used in the treatment of areas around the eye, for drooping eyelids, for the treatment of cellulite, as well as on the cheekbones and forehead.

The results of radio frequency treatments tend to be accumulative and vary according to the areas of the body that are being treated and the body's responsiveness to it. Optimal results tend to be achieved after an average period of approximately six months, and the results tend to last for three years. A key advantage of these treatments is that they tend to achieve very natural results. For optimal results, radio frequency treatments tend to be used in conjunction with other treatments, such as injections of hyaluronic acid. Among the advantages of radio frequency treatments is that there is limited to no downtime, and side effects are typically no more severe than some redness for a few hours after the procedure.

Infrared light and bi-polar radio frequency treatments can also be used for skin tightening. These treatments are designed to stimulate the production of collagen, which in turn, promotes the tightening of the skin. These treatments are often successful in the treatment of loose skin and sagginess of the face and neck, and the texture of the skin is also smoothed by the tightening and firming effects of the treatment. These procedures are not invasive, there is no recovery time, and most clients experience only mild redness immediately after treatment. Results can be noticed immediately after the procedure, and a gradual improvement in the skin's firmness, tightness, and texture is achieved as your skin's collagen increases. Approximately three to five sessions at three- to four-week intervals are required, and follow-up treatments are recommended either once or twice per year.

Nano Ablative Lasers

The nano ablative laser is a fast and effective laser treatment that is designed to improve skin texture and decrease the appearance of fine lines and wrinkles, leaving you with a fresh complexion and with minimal downtime.

This type of laser immediately removes the layers of the epidermis using light energy, and it has the precision to remove layers of skin to specific areas and to the desired depth. This type of laser treatment is considered to be safer than microdermabrasion and chemical peels, which cannot reach the desired depth safely.

Not only does this laser remove the outer-most layers of the skin, it also heats up the epidermis. This heat stimulates collagen production in the dermal layers, which over time plumps the skin and reduces the appearance of fine lines and wrinkles. The heat of the laser also has a tightening effect, and optimal results are usually achieved between four to six weeks.

Nano ablative lasers are a quick and effective resurfacing treatment, but they can cause some side effects, including infection, hyperpigmentation, as well as redness and swelling. Contraindications for the treatment include women who are pregnant or breast feeding, the presence of metal implants in the skin, an active skin infection, keloids, as well as taking acne medications within the past year.

Photofacials (IPL)

The intense pulsed-light photofacial (also called IPL) uses high-energy light on the skin to treat pigmentation problems, such as dark spots, spider veins, or facial redness. This treatment uses a non-ablative laser that is designed not to damage the upper layers of the skin in the same way that other laser treatments do. This device damages the lower layers of the skin in a controlled manner, which then stimulates the production of collagen.

Although photofacials can be very effective, the treatment can be quite painful, so a numbing agent of a local anesthetic is sometimes used by skin specialists.

For best results, five treatments are conducted every two weeks. Thereafter, maintenance treatments may be required every six to twelve months.

Radiofrequency Treatments

Radiofrequency treatments are generally used for skin tightening at both the superficial level and the sub-dermal skin layer. The result is the stimulation of elastin production and new elastin synthesis, which results in the long-term treatment of superficial wrinkles, and a firmer, more youthful appearance. There are two types of radiofrequency treatment procedures, which are monopolar and bipolar. In these treatments, radiofrequency currents are targeted into the skin in a controlled manner, which in turn, promotes collagen production. This treatment requires no downtime and the most common side effect is facial redness immediately after the procedure.

Infared and Personal LED Treatments

The most commonly used LED lights (light-emitting diode) in dermatology are infrared, amber, red, and blue. Amber light is promotes new collagen and elastin, red promotes circulation and reduces inflammation, blue destroys acne-causing bacteria, and infrared accelerates the skin recovery process. These different lights are often combined, but any of these treatments can be used in isolation to target specific issues.

LED treatments work by channelling light waves deep into the skin and by triggering intracellular reactions. For instance, with the red LED, the skin responds by building, strengthening, and maximizing the skin's cellular structure. In addition, red laser treatments target the oil glands to reduce cytokines, which are thought to cause some types of chronic acne.

Among the benefits of LED treatments is that the light doesn't actually heat the skin, and therefore no thermal damage is sustained. Also, unlike lasers and acid peels, there is no removal of skin. Instead, the light works on your skin painlessly.

LED light therapy builds collagen in quantifiable percentages and corrects surface damage, such as sun damage, large pores, and wrinkles. In the past, these were skin conditions that could only be treated with a laser or chemical peel, but LED light treatments have really revolutionized non-invasive dermatology treatments.

Combining Radiofrequency Treatments with Other Treatments

Radio frequency and IPL can work synergistically to produce smoother, tighter skin, as well as long-term mild wrinkle reduction. The combination of the two treatments helps overall appearnce o appearance of skin discoloration and texture. Radio frequency following Lipodissolve significantly improves skin smoothness and prevents texture irregularities after fat removal (commn comoon common complaints for many who use some fat dissloving procedures). Another benefit of Radio Frequency is it's ability to accerlaacclerate accelerate applied after an ultrasound fat reduction procedure can accelerate lymphatic drainage of fat, after lipposolve treatments which contributes to improves skin tightness and its overall appearance.

Radio frequency treatment takes no longer than approximately 20-45 minutes for most treatments areas. Although some effects are visible after just one session, an average of four to eight weekly skin-tightening treatments is recommended for optimal results.

Chemical Peels

A chemical peel involves the controlled application of toxic chemicals directly to the skin to produce tissue death. The depth of the wound inflicted by the chemical is dependent on the condition that is being treated. After the peel, the damaged skin regenerates, which produces a more youthful and smooth appearance. Chemical peels are categorized by the depth of damage that they inflict on the skin: As the name suggests, superficial peels do not damage tissue below the skin's most superficial layer; medium peels generally reach the superficial layer of the dermis while deep peels are designed to target the deeper layers of the skin's dermis. Common chemicals in peeling treatments are retinoids, alpha-hydroxy acids, and beta-hydroxy acids. Chemical peels are used for sun-damaged skin and uneven pigmentation, and they can also be used to treat acne scarring.

Patients who have dark pigmented skin should be very cautious about chemical peels because hyperpigmentation (darkening of the skin)and hypopigmentation (lightening of skin) can occur when the skin heals. Other risks of chemical peels are scarring and infection, however very uncommon especially o if when performed under the care of a trained provider of and facility. Also, the skin is particularly sensitive after this procedure, so sun avoidance is critical during the healing process. Last important note to mention, discontinue all retinol and glycolic skincare products3-5 days prior to your treatment.

Microdermabrasion

Microdermabrasion is a machine-assisted skin-exfoliating treatment. Microdermabrasion is a painless, noninvasive skin-rejuvenation procedure that applies a combination of a fine abrasive crystals and vacuum suction onto the skin. The procedure takes approximately 30-60 minutes, with no downtime. The process of microdermabrasion works by removing the top few layers of the skin. Because the treatment is quite superficial, improvements in the skin tend to be only temporary, and multiple treatments are required for optimal results.

Microdermabrasion has the advantage of being a low-risk procedure, and it has minimal downtime compared with some of the other more invasive resurfacing methods, such as dermabrasion and chemical peeling. Since microdermabrasion removes only the most superficial layers of the skin, it is better suited for mild and superficial issues, such as early photoaging, fine lines, age spots, acne, and superficial scarring, although the results are not dramatic. Although the face is the most common area for microdermabrasion, any skin area, including the neck, chest, back, and hands can be treated. It can also be useful for treating mild and superficial skin conditions, including minor scarring, minor discoloration, and fine lines; however, it is not effective for deeper wrinkles, more severe scars, skin sagging, or general loss of elasticity. With so many other noninvasive treatments available these days, microdermabrasion is often used to treat post-procedure via total exfoliation.

Microneedling and PRP

The advantages of using platelet-rich plasma (PRP) for aesthetic medicine are tissue regeneration, rejuvenation, and recruitment of other cells to the site of injury, and an increase in collagen production, which can increase skin thickness and overall skin health.

PRP has been used to treat acne, scarring, and alopecia, but it is also effective for skin rejuvenation and tightening around the eyes (for thin crepe-like skin and fine lines) and for the cheeks, mid-face, neck, throat, jawline, and the back of hands.

Platelet-rich plasma is injected by multiple tiny punctures under the dermis, with or without topical local anesthesia. When PRP is injected into the damaged area, it stimulates the tissue, causing mild inflammation that triggers the healing process. As a result, new collagen develops, and as this new collagen matures, it begins to shrink, which tightens and strengthens the skin. Improvements in skin texture and tone are generally noticeable within three weeks though collagen regeneration typically takes approximately three months.

PRP can be used in conjunction with skincare and light treatments for optimal results. Treatment results vary but can last up to 18 months for most patients, and biannual treatments will help to maintain results. PRP contains beneficial growth factors, and accordingly, it can also be used to re-plump areas of lost volume or scarring.

The latest facial rejuvenation procedure is the PRP facelift which combines the power PRP and facial fillers being injected to minimize the appearance of facial aging. This non-surgical procedure promotes new tissue growth to improve overall facial skin tone for a more youthful appearance. The PRP is combined with a facial filler and then re-injected into targeting areas of the face. There is minimal downtime from this procedure. It often leads to brighter healthier looking skin and colle collagen stimulation. There is always a risk of bruising when ned needles are involved but avoiding blood thinning ing product medication medications and supplements help.

The appearance of a facial lift can be achieved using a combination of fillers along with PRP. The fillers provide an instant fill or volume correction while the PRP initiates a skin regeneration process. The use of PRP and fillers in combination both enhances the skin tone and texture, and it also prolongs the filler correction for approximately three to six months longer than if the filler was used alone.

PRP in combination with fractional ablative/nano ablative lasers for deep wrinkles and severe photodamaged skin has also been shown to yield good results because functional laser treatments are known for their ability to retexture skin. Following your laser treatment, activated PRP serum is applied to the skin by an automatic microneedle. This microneedling inserts minute wounds into the skin. These wounds take in the PRP serum, which initiates collagen production and tissue enhancement from growth factors found in the plasma serum. While it is still a relatively new procedure, microneedling is also producing impressive treatment results for scarring and stretch marks.

Nevertheless, patients who do not want adjunctive treatments can still benefit from PRP. The activated PRP serum can be injected just under the skin surface to stimulate the body to produce its own filler via its own collagen production, and while this will not yield the same results as a filler, some textural improvements are nonetheless likely.

Noninvasive Fat-Removal Procedures

CoolSculpting, Vanquish, and TruSculpt

CoolSculpting is an FDA-approved technique for fat reduction, which freezes fat in specific areas. It is a non-invasive procedure that does not require the use of anesthesia. The device functions a bit like a vacuum in that it draws in the tissue between the cooling panels. The applicator is then removed and is massaged briefly by the physician. Over a period of several months, the fat cells that have been frozen are naturally excreted via the body's metabolic processes. Results are quite good, and patients can generally expect to lose about 20 percent of the fat in the targeted area. For optimal results, the procedure can be repeated. Due to the vacuum, not all patients are suitable candidates for this treatment. A patient's BMI (body mass index) needs to be taken into account because if the patient's BMI is too high, the suction may not attach, which renders the treatment impossible. Pricing is usually based on the hand-piece used and the treatment area. For example, a patient who has a large torso may require 2 to 3 applicators to treat the abdominal area.

Vanquish is another non-surgical fat-reduction device that is FDA-approved for tissue heating. Rather than freezing the fat,

Vanquish utilizes radio frequency to heat and remove fat. Unlike CoolSculpting, in which the applicator comes in direct contact with the skin, the patient lies under the device while the sensors read the body fat to determine the energy level of needed to target specific areas. The hand-piece covers and treats the entire abdomen and love handles in one session. The treatment takes an average of 30 to 45 minutes, and patients typically have four sessions at weekly intervals. As is the case with CoolSculpting, the fat cells are then eliminated by the body naturally. Approximately 60 percent reduction in fat in the targeted area is achieved with Vanquish, and also, Vanquish tends to produce faster results than CoolSculpting. Unlike other body-sculpting machines that kill fat cells, Vanquish also improves skin tightening.

TruSculpt is an additional non-invasive fat-reducing treatment that can help to contour, smooth, and tighten areas of the body. To break up fat cells in targeted areas of the body, the radio-frequency energy enters the skin and travels towards the underlying fat tissue. Since the fat tissue is specifically targeted, the energy does not affect other bodily tissue. The treatment causes the fat cells to self-destruct, and these fat cells are then flushed from the system via the body's own lymphatic process. The procedure is a good alternative to liposuction, and optimal results are generally achieved after three months of treatment.

Kybella

Some people develop a double chin when they age, despite weight loss and exercise to improve muscle tone. A double chin can result from aging or genetic factors, which renders it difficult to treat with diet and exercise. Until relatively recently, the main treatment option for a double chin and fat deposits was invasive liposuction, which involves risks and significant downtime. Kybella is the first injection approved in the United States to dissolve fat cells, and it offers a non-surgical means of treating double chins, which involves a series of fat-dissolving injections. Kybella is administered via a series of fast and pain-free injections, and within a few months, the double chin diminishes leaving you with a more defined and youthful chin and neck. Kybella is a naturally-occurring molecule in the body that aids in the breakdown of dietary fat, and when it is injected into the fat below the chin, it ruptures the fat cell membranes and permanently destroys chin fat. Up to six treatments might be required to achieve optimal results, and treatments should be administered at intervals of no less than one month. The treatment typically takes less than 30 minutes, and recovery time is minimal. The treatment does not require any maintenance because destruction of fat cells is permanent.

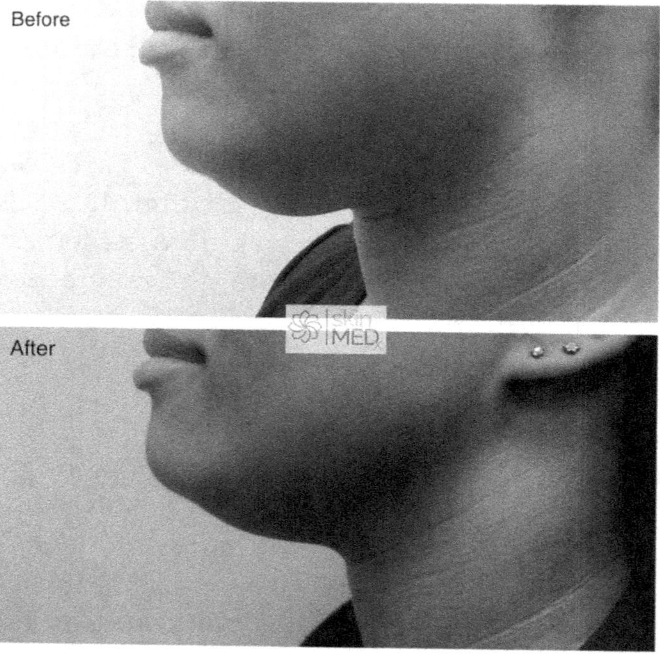

Other facial areas, such as jowls, can potentially also benefit from Kybella injections for small fat reductions. As we age, the skin and any underlying fat drifts down over the jawline, which creates jowls and increased lower facial width. While fat reduction alone is usually insufficient to treat jowls in most patients, it is one component of treatment that can help to produce an overall better result when used in conjunction with other treatments, such as fillers. Treatment for jowls works in much the same way as the treatment of chin fat, and two to three sessions might be required for optimal results. Considerable swelling after the injections is expected during the first week.

While Kybella is predominantly used to treat chin fat and jowls, it can be used on virtually any part of the body. Accordingly, it is becoming increasingly popular in the treatment of bra fat, stomach fat, and buttocks rolls. For treatment in each of these areas, Kybella requires multiple treatments, depending on the amount of fat being targeted, but the average amount of sessions for small- to moderate-sized fat rolls is two to three. Typical side effects of this treatment on the body include bruising and slight swelling, but these tend to only last a maximum of two weeks.

Take Charge of Your Beauty

CHAPTER NINE

Common Questions

How Do I Get Rid of Wrinkles under My Eyes?

The first recommendation is to address the eyes using Botox. Nevertheless, Botox cannot treat the deeper lines that go all the way in towards the nose. For deeper lines, you should consider laser resurfacing, ablative and non-ablative treatments, microneedling with PRP, and radio frequency treatments. Dermal fillers can sometimes help as well. Although this book is about non-invasive treatments, in some cases, deep lines that are accompanied by excessive skin tissue are best treated with minor surgery. In some cases adding a filler in the eye area is simply not the best decision if extreme laxity is the issue above or below the eyelids. In these cases, I refer patients to a local plastic surgeon for a minor, in-office procedure called blepharoplasty. An important caveat with all of these treatments is that a skin specialist needs to assess your own individual anatomy before a suitable treatment is selected for you.

My Eyes Are Sunken. What Are My Options?

Sunken eyes are best addressed using dermal fillers. Often the filler will be placed in the cheek area to help restore the fat deposits in the cheeks that have fallen. In the process of adding volume, the appearance of sunken eyes may be improved, but sometimes treating the lower lids with fillers called "tear troughs" can produce better results.

I Have a Bump in My Nose, But I Don't Want to Have a Nose Job. Are There Other Options?

When we think "nose job," we generally think of a surgical procedure whereby the structure of the nose is changed. The change can involve the addition or subtraction of bone or cartilage (invasive surgery), or it might involve grafting of tissue from another part of the body or implanting synthetic material to alter the shape of the nose (non-invasive treatment). This noninvasive treatment can be referred to as nose moulding, or a "lunchtime nose job."

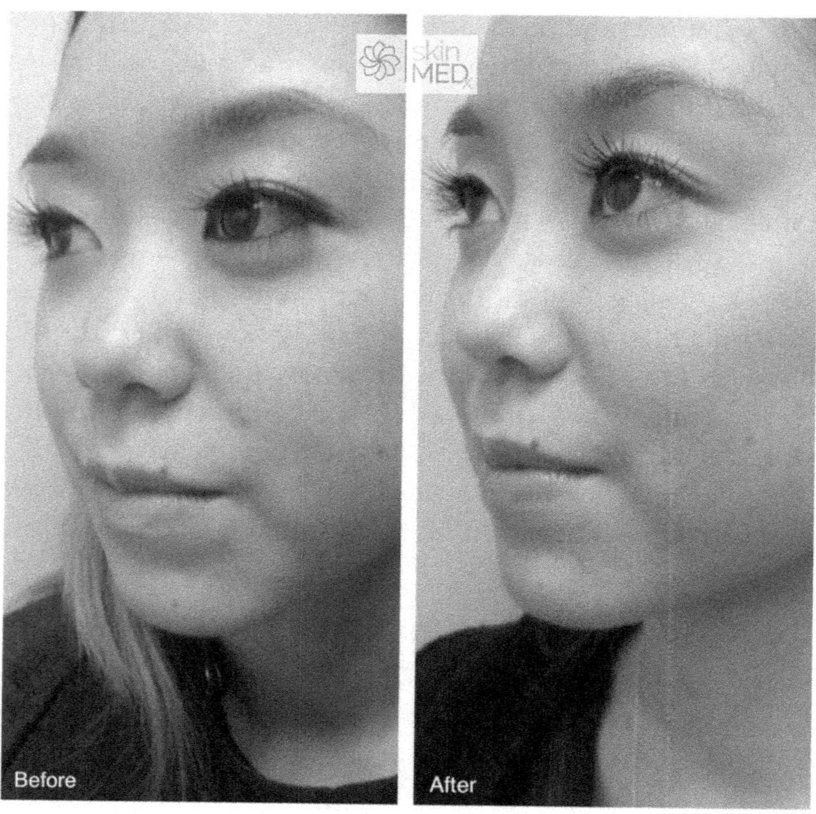

     Take Charge of Your Beauty

Remember we talked earlier about dermal fillers in chapter Five? Dermal fillers can produce some excellent results.

- If you have a smaller nose, you may want the filler injected into certain areas of the nose to make it appear larger and more defined. Alternatively, the angle or tip of the nose can be altered using fillers to improve its overall shape.
- Fillers can be used to fill out hollows or a depression in your nose to help with definition and improve your profile.
- Fillers can straighten a hook nose by filling in the area above and below the bend.
- If your nose is crooked, meaning it deviates slightly to one side, then fillers can make it appear straighter.
- It is very common to have this procedure to straighten out subtle humps and bumps and-or to elongate the wings of the nose.

This procedure is not suitable for everyone, nor will it always achieve the results you are hoping for. For instance, if you have more prominent or obvious nose irregularities, such as an oversized nose or a nose that has large bumps, then fillers might not be your best option. Conversely, if surgery is not for you, or you simply want to see how your nose would look if you had a surgical procedure, then fillers are a good impermanent solution.

I Have Smokers' Lines, But I Have Never Smoked—Help!

Smokers' lines are a combination of lack of laxity and lack of musculature supporting the orbicularis muscle. They are common with age. As we age, we often see changes in the lips—the lips seem to shrink and fall inwards and lip lines develop around the mouth. A few things can be done to treat the lips. To start, I recommend

Botox for some people to relax the muscles that are contributing to the lines around the mouth. Also, fillers with HA can help reform the foundations around the structure of the mouth, and lasers can also help (preferably ablative lasers). Fillers can be added into the lips, which can help stop lipstick bleeding into the fine lines of the lips, and these will also restore your volume. Often patients imagine they will have over-sized lips, but as discussed in chapter Five, there are many different fillers, and they all differ in terms of how they work and how they are used. For example, some fillers can add hydration and shape and very little volume, while other fillers can add a lot more volume. The choice of treatment depends on the skin specialist's assessment of the patient, what the patient wants, as well as face balance and symmetry.

My Hands Look So Old. Can You Make Them More Youthful?

Hands can prematurely age due to sun damage and loss of elasticity. A few things can be done to improve the appearance of the hands. You can treat sunspots with brightening creams, or alternatively, a photofacial (IPL) treatment can be done to remove brown spots and redness. If you wish to achieve skin tightening on the hands, then an ablative treatment might be more effective. Maintenance treatments, such as microneedling and platelet rich plasma (PRP), are also effective for stimulating collagen production. The best treatment for very prominent veins in the hands is putting fillers in the hands. Hand fillers generally only require between three to five injections per hand, and the process is very quick. I always advise there is a risk of minimal swelling for a couple of days, but the end result is invariably very pleasing to my patients. Results can last up to two years.

Hollow Temples—What Can I Do?

I am noticing hollow temples are becoming more prevalent, especially in patients after I have done mid-face volumizing. Putting extra volume in the mid-face can sometimes accentuate the natural hollowing of the temples that affects many people as they age. I often also see hollow temples with runners. I usually recommend dermal fillers to treat this issue. An important precaution with this filler as well as other fillers is that it needs to be injected by a skin specialist who is both skilled and experienced because it is often a challenge for even experienced skin specialists to treat this area.

My Earlobes Look So Saggy and Old —What Are My Options?

This is common after years of wearing especially large and heavy earrings, but it can happen during the natural aging process. Small amounts of filler can placed in the earlobe to bring it back to life. You can go back to wearing your large hoop earrings!

My Chest Looks Older Than My Face —What Can Be Done?

Most women focus primarily on the care of their face when it comes to prevention and protection because it is the first place we start to see the early signs of aging. However, the neck, chest, and hands are often neglected when it comes to sun protection. The sun damage and natural aging process leave behind crepey skin, discoloration, and poor skin quality.

I always recommend prevention: It is never too late for sun protection and sun damage prevention. Once the damage has occurred, there are a number of options. I often find that the chest is the most badly affected by sun damage, and in some cases, there are signs of either skin cancer or pre-skin cancer. Sun damage on the chest often presents as discoloration of the skin and scaly or rough patches. Therefore, the first line of treatment should be to treat the sun damage: Have your skincare provider treat any skin cancers first before you look at treating the cosmetic side of things.

For the chest area, some of the cosmetic options are topical creams with retinols, brightening products, and glycolic acids. The most common treatment for these areas starts with photofacials (or IPL for the discoloration). For crepey skin, microneedling or PRP (vampire facial) can be used, and ablative treatments and radio frequency are also options.

Is It Possible to Treat Neck Lines?

Botox is a great option to soften necklines. Sometimes after Botox is completed, fine fillers can be injected into the vertical lines of the neck. Laser should also be considered if your skin specialist uses laser to treat your face, because you can often get a discount price if you choose to have both your face and neck treated with lasers.

What Can Be Done to Treat Jowls?

The upper face is usually treated with fillers to add volume and to help lift the fat pads that have fallen and which contribute to the nasolabial and marionette folds around the mouth (smile lines). Every face requires an individualized consultation. Treatment for this area often involves a few different treatments, including the use of fillers and neuomodulators, and sometimes skin-tightening devices. Although not currently FDA-approved for the treatment of jowls, Kybella injections into the fat are a new and effective option. Again, all of these procedures must be done by a highly-experienced skin specialist due to risk of nerve irritation. Although not permanent, swelling can affect the nerve, cause some discomfort, and change the shape of the smile.

What Is a "Blepharoplasty"?

Blepharoplasty is a medical term for eyelid surgery of the upper or lower eyelid. The effects typically last anywhere between 5 and 10 years. As with any other procedure, there are risks, which include post-surgical complications. There are no other medical alternatives to blepharoplasty that can reshape your eyelids.

Blepharoplasty corrects heavy or over-hanging upper eyelids, fat deposits, excess tissue, or in some cases, muscles, to improve the appearance of the eyes. As we age, some of us experience a degree of sagging and excess skin surrounding the eyes, which over time, can become so extensive that it affects your range of vision. If this is the case, then the procedure serves a functional rather than a purely cosmetic purpose. Other reasons for this procedure might be bags under the eyes, drooping eyes, or if you cannot apply eyelid makeup easily. If you have excess fatty deposits that create puffiness beneath the eyelid skin, droopiness of the lower eyelids, extra skin and fine wrinkles of the lower eyelid, then this treatment might be a good option for you.

Why Does Everyone Recommend Retinol?

Skincare specialists consider retinol the Holy Grail of skincare because of its impressive anti-aging properties. Retinol helps to reduce the appearance of fine lines, it evens out our complexions, and it also unclogs our pores.

As you may be aware, retinol is a form of vitamin A, and it works by boosting your collagen production, which as previously discussed, helps to keep your skin firm and elastic. Retinol also speeds up cellular turnover, which speeds up the renewal process.

Over time, it reduces the appearance of wrinkles and dark spots, and it brightens the complexion. It can also be used in the treatment of acne. Nevertheless, using retinol too much can irritate your skin.

So, how much retinol should you use? To answer that as simply as possible, it comes down to your skin's needs, skin type, concerns, conditions, and your skin's tolerance to retinol. Determining your skin's tolerance to retinol will come down to trial and error. You should experiment with different formulations, strengths, and application methods, and you should also monitor your skin's response. It is easy to get carried away with a product like this, so just keep in mind that not everyone's skin can tolerate these products in higher concentrations.

That does not mean you would not see incredible benefits using a product with a lower concentration of retinol and by using it daily. So, if you have uneven skin tone, loss of firmness, and deeper wrinkles, then a moderate product might work well if it is applied two to three times per week. As mentioned, the frequency of use depends on your skin and how it responds. Again, your skincare specialist is the best person to consult for advice about the best retinol products for your skin.

Why Can't Botox Help?

Botox only works for smoothing out lines and preventing them from becoming more pronounced. It does not do anything for sun-damaged skin or lines caused by skin sagging, such as nasolabial folds. Botox injections are effective in treating some muscle-pull creases, but not all of them, and also the results are temporary. The injections will not improve the overall quality of the skin, such as texture changes or uneven pigmentation. Treatment options for improving the quality of the skin include laser resurfacing, fillers, microneedling, etc. Botox injections will not improve sagging and redundant skin. Lifting procedures are necessary for these conditions. Nevertheless, Botox is often used in combination with other treatments, such as fillers. A combination of these injectables can yield better results than either of these treatments used in isolation.

Take Charge of Your Beauty

CHAPTER TEN

The Future of Aesthetics

The exciting thing about the world of dermatological aesthetics is that it is constantly evolving with advances in technology, ongoing research, and the very promising results of clinical trials. While there is no "one size fits all" miracle treatment, the most cutting-edge techniques in the world of aesthetics are producing unprecedented results that are showing promise in stripping away the years.

With that said, dermatology is becoming more about prevention. I am seeing greater numbers of patients in their twenties who are seeking treatments to help them preserve their youth because prevention really is the most effective way to maintain a youthful appearance. From small amounts of Botox, to prescription skincare, these young people are leaving nothing to chance. Also, with the ever-increasing affordability of non-invasive dermatology, not to mention the ever-developing technologies that are giving rise to more effective and longer-lasting results, the world of aesthetics continues to gather interest from people from all walks of life.

In the past, the concept of facial rejuvenation was dominated by invasive surgical procedures, such as facelifts and liposuction surgeries. Nevertheless, the future of aesthetics is evolving towards increasingly simpler and less invasive procedures that impose hardly any disruption and require minimal (if any) downtime. The market continues to introduce new technologies that provide effective, safe, relatively long-lasting, and natural results. While there is no doubt that the popular surgical and non-surgical procedures, such as rhinoplasty, will continue to maintain an important role in rejuvenation, Botox, new types of fillers, and soft-tissue augmentation represent an important nonsurgical resource that, combined with traditional techniques, can improve or extend results.

The Future of Energy Treatments

While energy-based treatments, such as lasers, have demonstrated efficacy in treating a variety of skin conditions, these treatments have traditionally been used to target the blood and water in the skin. However, a new generation of treatments might discover technologies that can target the lipids, which are contained in the sebaceous glands, and if that is the case, future treatments for acne might be a laser that is more selective in treating acne via targeting the skin's lipids than the current technologies. At present, technologies that specifically target acne are in the very early stages of development, but they will dramatically change the way that acne is currently treated. In addition, the arrival of more lasers that produce less downtime and greater accessibility to these treatments for all patients with different skin types appear to be on the horizon of future cosmetic dermatology.

The Future of Fat-Reduction Treatments

The latest research is focusing on the improvement of existing devices that use targeted energy sources to remove fat and cellulite. The fat-reduction treatments that are currently on the market include CoolSculpting, Vanquish ME, and TruSculpt, among others, which either freeze or melt fat. Although current treatments are popular and showing good results, research is investigating what sorts of improvements can be made in future. With the high demand of these treatments, there is no doubt it will be a growing niche in the industry.

In addition, lipid-targeting wavelengths might facilitate the use of noninvasive fat treatments while fat-reducing lasers might be used to supplement the CoolSculpting procedure that freezes off fat. Kybella is a revolutionary treatment in the world of noninvasive body scultpting, with thanks to the clever innovation of Dr. Michael Kolodney and Dr. Adam Rotunda who co-invented Kybella. Although Kybella was originally approved for the treatment of chin fat, it is currently being applied in the treatment of jowls as well as in the removal of stomach fat, bra fat, and buttocks fat. A possible evolution of this technology is combining it with ultrasound, or alternatively, combining radio-frequency energy with ultrasound for optimal results that not only eliminate fat, but also help with skin tightening.

Innovation in Topical Skin Product Delivery

In coming years, the trend toward less invasive technologies is likely to continue not only in facial treatments, fat removal, and body-sculpting treatments, but also in new, more efficient means of delivering a variety of drugs into the body. For instance, some of the most promising future technologies involve using fractional lasers to inject drugs into the body via the skin. This research is still in its infancy although it does pose some exciting possibilities for the future of noninvasive dermatology. In similar research, dermatologists are currently investigating the possibility of delivering skin lightening agents and other topical skin products via a blative fractional resurfacing . Over-the-counter agents, such as hyaluronic acid for skin rejuvenation and skin-lightening ingredients, such as vitamin C, might well be the way forward. Furthermore, an additional possibility is that refraction technology might be used for the delivery of growth factors and other wound-healing agents; this technology would potentially deliver growth factors with greater efficiency than is currently possible topically.

The Future of Sun Protection

Asian sunscreens are among the best in the world. For example, on Japanese sunscreens is an additional label called the Japanese Persistent Pigment Darkening (PPD) designation, which is used by many Asian brands to provide a more detailed UV rating. "The PA+ to +++" rating indicates how much UVA protection that you get from the product, and the number of plus symbols after the "PA" refers to the amount of UVA protection you get from a product. Three pluses is the highest level of protection, while two and three pluses provide only moderate and minimal protection, respectively.

In the US, there are currently no regulations in regards to the amount of UVA protection you can get in American sunscreens. As discussed in chapter Three, photoaging is one of the most significant contributors of aging, so although protection from UVB rays is important, you also need to consider UVA protection to prevent premature lines and spots caused by sun damage. UVA filter ingredients, such as tinosorb and mexoryl, are used as UVA blockers in Asian and European formulations, but these products are not yet available in the US. Therefore, it would seem that future advancements in sun protection within the US are much needed to address the pervasive effects of premature aging caused by UVA radiation.

There has been increasing interest in medications that claim to protect against sun damage, but the results with most products that have been tested have been disappointing. Nevertheless, Heliocare Oral is the first oral sun protectant that has a clinically demonstrated capacity to prevent free radicals, reduce premature aging, as well as minimize hyperpigmentation caused by sun damage. The product ingredients are beta-carotene, green tea, and a natural fern extract, and the product is taken orally in tablet-form.

In fact, Heliocare Oral has been extensively researched now for over ten years, and the results are promising. It is a product that is being widely recommended by skin specialists.

The research that has been done to date suggests that Heliocare Oral can protect the skin from sun damage, which can lead to skin cancer. Heliocare Oral enters your blood stream and works from the inside out, as opposed to sunscreen which works from the outside in. Nevertheless, the research cautions that other sun protection measures should be used with products like these, including sunscreens, protective clothing, and avoiding the sun during the hottest part of the day. While Heliocare Oral is an important innovation, ongoing research continues on oral products and other technologies that can potentially be used to minimize the harmful impacts of UVA and UVB radiation. I anticipate that these new technologies are likely to give rise to an approach that leans more heavily towards prevention.

Noninvasive Advancements in Vaginal Rejuvenation

I have a number of women patients who have suffered from the effects of childbirth, the aging process, menopause, and chemotherapy. Until recently, the only option for treatments in this area required invasive and potentially traumatic surgeries that carried extended downtimes.

In 2017, women have options in regards to non-surgical procedures that address their concerns about intimate health, and with minimal downtown and discomfort.

Promising developments in laser treatment have given rise to treatments that address symptoms related to vaginal wellness and appearance, such as changes associated with childbirth, trauma, illness, and aging.

After childbirth, some women experience loosening of the vaginal canal while menopausal and post-menopausal women can experience vulvo vaginal atrophy, which can produce symptoms of burning, dryness, and discomfort. Most commonly, women suffer from urinary incontinence post-pregnancy and after menopause. As women age, they might also experience cosmetic changes to their genitalia, such as pigmentation and sagging. These are all becoming more common discussions in dermatology settings and women are seeking treatments!

Laser treatments can deliver controlled energy to the vaginal tissue to stimulate the produce of collagen, which in turn, improves skin tone, texture, and appearance. In addition, the laser stimulates a healing response that initiates remodeling of the tissue fibers, and this serves to restore flexibility and shape while also enhancing moisture to optimal levels in the vaginal canal.

The Only Thing That Is Certain Is Change

The only thing that is certain in life is change, so it is important to keep an eye on the ways in which the medical aesthetics industry is evolving. You might not want to look at face-enhancing procedures or body rejuvenation just yet, but it's useful to understand why some people are choosing to do so. Nobody ever had too much information about the future of their bodies, so it pays to consider the future.

Some Final Thoughts on Inner and Outer Beauty

Inner beauty reflects on the outer beauty. For instance, if you look at any child from anywhere in the world, there is subtle beauty in them: They don't require cosmetics to enhance their beauty because it's their innocence, honesty, and uninhibitedness that truly enhances their youthful beauty. Societal perceptions about physical beauty are forever evolving, and while physical features are largely heritable, they can be enhanced or minimized using cosmetics as well as invasive and noninvasive cosmetic procedures. Nevertheless, outer beauty is what originally draws people to each other. Outer beauty most certainly enhances inner beauty because it tends to make people more confident and at peace with themselves and others, which are traits that people are biologically primed to be attracted to. Nevertheless, inner beauty is the most enduring expression of beauty, and traits, such as kindness, humility, generosity, empathy, and patience, most certainly go a long way towards enhancing a person's overall beauty. These features cannot be manufactured, and people who are happy within themselves and who possess inner beauty tend to have a genuine passion for life that goes beyond the material world of appearances and possessions. Inner beauty does not fade with age; in fact, it often grows as a person ages and gains wisdom.

As a skin specialist, it is a great honor and privilege to be able to assist my patients to bring out their inner beauty by restoring their outer beauty. The two work together synergistically because it is a person's outer beauty that originally draws people to them. So, via enhancing outer beauty, and by doing so enhancing their inner beauty, these two types of beauty can help a person to be more successful with first impressions, secure jobs, improve their social status, nurture their friendships, and generally enjoy a better quality of life.

Linda Rank

Take Charge of Your Beauty